Somatoform and Factitious Disorders

Review of Psychiatry Series
John M. Oldham, M.D.
Michelle B. Riba, M.D., M.S.
Series Editors

Somatoform and Factitious Disorders

EDITED BY

Katharine A. Phillips, M.D.

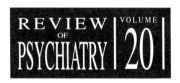

No. 3

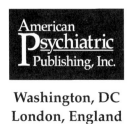

Washington, DC
London, England

American Psychiatric Publishing, Inc.
1400 K Street, NW
Washington, DC 20005
www.appi.org

The correct citation for this book is

Phillips KA (editor): *Somatoform and Factitious Disorders* (Review of Psychiatry Series, Volume 20, Number 3; Oldham JM and Riba MB, series editors). Washington, DC, American Psychiatric Publishing, 2001

Library of Congress Cataloging-in-Publication Data
Somatoform and factitious disorders / edited by Katharine A. Phillips.
        p. cm. — (Review of psychiatry ; v. 20, no. 3)
    Includes bibliographical references and index.
    ISBN 1-58562-029-7 (alk. paper)
    1. Somatoform disorders. 2. Factitious disorders. 3. Medicine, Psychosomatic.
    I. Phillips, Katharine A. II. Review of psychiatry series ; v. 20, 3
    [DNLM: 1. Somatoform Disorders. 2. Factitious Disorders. WM 170 S6927 2001]
    RC552.S66 .S676 2001
    616.89—dc21

                                                                00-067403

British Library Cataloguing in Publication Data
A CIP record is available from the British Library.

Contents

Contributors

Holly N. Deemer, M.A.
Doctoral Candidate in Clinical Psychology, Department of Psychology, University of Alabama, Tuscaloosa, Alabama

Brian A. Fallon, M.D.
Associate Professor of Clinical Psychiatry, Columbia University College of Physicians and Surgeons, New York, New York; Director, Somatic Disorders Treatment Program, New York State Psychiatric Institute, New York, New York

Suzanne Feinstein, Ph.D.
Research Psychologist, New York State Psychiatric Institute, New York, New York

Marc D. Feldman, M.D.
CPM Medical Director; Vice Chair, Clinical Services; and Associate Professor, Department of Psychiatry and Behavioral Neurobiology, University of Alabama at Birmingham, Birmingham, Alabama

James C. Hamilton, Ph.D.
Assistant Professor, Department of Psychology, University of Alabama, Tuscaloosa, Alabama

Vicenzio Holder-Perkins, M.D.
Instructor, Department of Psychiatry, Georgetown University School of Medicine, Washington, D.C.; Instructor, Department of Psychiatry, George Washington University School of Medicine, Washington, D.C.

José R. Maldonado, M.D.
Assistant Professor of Psychiatry; Medical Director, Consultation/Liaison Psychiatry; and Chief, Medical and Forensic Psychiatry, Department of Psychiatry and Behavioral Sciences, Stanford University School of Medicine, Stanford, California

John M. Oldham, M.D.
Dollard Professor and Acting Chairman, Department of Psychiatry, Columbia University College of Physicians and Surgeons, New York, New York

Katharine A. Phillips, M.D.
Associate Professor of Psychiatry and Human Behavior, Brown University School of Medicine, Providence, Rhode Island; Associate Medical Director, Ambulatory Care, and Director, Body Dysmorphic Disorder Program, Butler Hospital, Providence, Rhode Island

Michelle B. Riba, M.D., M.S.
Associate Chair for Education and Academic Affairs, Department of Psychiatry, University of Michigan Medical School, Ann Arbor, Michigan

David Spiegel, M.D.
Professor of Psychiatry; Director, Psychosocial Treatment Laboratory; and Director, Complementary Medicine Clinic, Department of Psychiatry and Behavioral Sciences, Stanford University School of Medicine, Stanford, California

Thomas N. Wise, M.D.
Professor, Department of Psychiatry, Georgetown University School of Medicine, Washington, D.C.; Professor, Department of Psychiatry, Johns Hopkins University School of Medicine, Baltimore, Maryland; Medical Director, Behavioral Services, Inova Health Systems, Falls Church, Virginia

Introduction to the Review of Psychiatry Series

John M. Oldham, M.D., and
Michelle B. Riba, M.D., M.S., Series Editors

2001 Review of Psychiatry Series Titles

- *PTSD in Children and Adolescents*
  Edited by Spencer Eth, M.D.
- *Integrated Treatment of Psychiatric Disorders*
  Edited by Jerald Kay, M.D.
- *Somatoform and Factitious Disorders*
  Edited by Katharine A. Phillips, M.D.
- *Treatment of Recurrent Depression*
  Edited by John F. Greden, M.D.
- *Advances in Brain Imaging*
  Edited by John M. Morihisa, M.D.

In today's rapidly changing world, the dissemination of information is one of its rapidly changing elements. Information virtually assaults us, and proclaimed experts abound. Witness, for example, the 2000 presidential election in the United States, during which instant opinions were plentiful about the previously obscure science of voting machines, the electoral college, and the meaning of the words of the highest court in the land. For medicine the situation is the same: the World Wide Web virtually bulges with health advice, treatment recommendations, and strident warnings about the dangers of this approach or that. Authoritative and reliable guides to help the consumer differentiate between sound advice and unsubstantiated opinion are hard to come by, and our patients and their families may be misled by bad information without even knowing it.

At no time has it been more important, then, for psychiatrists and other clinicians to be well informed, armed with the very latest findings, and well versed in evidence-based medicine. We have designed Volume 20 of the Review of Psychiatry Series with these trends in mind—to be, if you will, a how-to manual: how to accurately identify illnesses, how to understand where they come from and what is going wrong in specific conditions, how to measure the extent of the problem, and how to design the best treatment, especially for the particularly difficult-to-treat disorders.

The central importance of stress as a pathogen in major mental illness throughout the life cycle is increasingly clear. One form of stress is *trauma.* Extreme trauma can lead to illness at any age, but its potential to set the stage badly for life when severe trauma occurs during early childhood is increasingly recognized. In *PTSD in Children and Adolescents,* Spencer Eth and colleagues review the evidence from animal and human studies of the aberrations, both psychological and biological, that can persist throughout adulthood as a result of trauma experienced during childhood. Newer technologies have led to new knowledge of the profound nature of some of these changes, from persistently altered stress hormones to gene expression and altered protein formation. In turn, hypersensitivities result from this early stress-induced biological programming, so that cognitive and emotional symptom patterns emerge rapidly in reaction to specific environmental stimuli.

Nowhere in the field of medicine is technology advancing more rapidly than in brain imaging, generating a level of excitement that surely surpasses the historical moment when the discovery of the X ray first allowed us to noninvasively see into the living human body. The new imaging methods, fortunately, do not involve the risk of radiation exposure, and the capacity of the newest imaging machines to reveal brain structure and function in great detail is remarkable. Yet in many ways these techniques still elude clinical application, since they are expensive and increasingly complex to administer and interpret. John Morihisa has gathered a group of our best experts to discuss the latest developments in *Advances in Brain Imaging,* and the shift toward greater clinical utility is clear in their descriptions of these methods. Perhaps most intriguing is the promise that through these methods we can identify, before the onset of symptoms, those most at risk of developing psychiatric disorders, as discussed by Daniel Pine regarding childhood disorders and by Harold Sackeim regarding late-life depression.

Certain conditions, such as the somatoform and factitious disorders, can baffle even our most experienced clinicians. As Katharine Phillips points out in her foreword to *Somatoform and Factitious Disorders*, these disorders frequently go unrecognized or are misdiagnosed, and patients with these conditions may be seen more often in the offices of nonpsychiatric physicians than in those of psychiatrists. Although these conditions have been reported throughout the recorded history of medicine, patients with these disorders either are fully convinced that their problems are "physical" instead of "mental" or choose to present their problems that way. In this book, experienced clinicians provide guidelines to help identify the presence of the somatoform and factitious disorders, as well as recommendations about their treatment.

Treatment of all psychiatric disorders is always evolving, based on new findings and clinical experience; at times, the field has become polarized, with advocates of one approach vying with advocates of another (e.g., psychotherapy versus pharmacotherapy). Patients, however, have the right to receive the best treatment available, and most of the time the best treatment includes psychotherapy *and* pharmacotherapy, as detailed in *Integrated Treatment of Psychiatric Disorders*. Jerald Kay and colleagues propose the term *integrated treatment* for this approach, a recommended fundamental of treatment planning. Psychotherapy alone, of course, may be the best treatment for some patients, just as pharmacotherapy may be the mainstay of treatment for others, but in all cases there should be thoughtful consideration of a combination of these approaches.

Finally, despite tremendous progress in the treatment of most psychiatric disorders, there are some conditions that are stubbornly persistent in spite of the best efforts of our experts. John Greden takes up one such area in *Treatment of Recurrent Depres-*

sion, referring to recurrent depression as one of the most disabling disorders of all, so that, in his opinion, "a call to arms" is needed. Experienced clinicians and researchers review optimal treatment approaches for this clinical population. As well, new strategies, such as vagus nerve stimulation and minimally invasive brain stimulation, are reviewed, indicating the need to go beyond our currently available treatments for these seriously ill patients.

All in all, we believe that Volume 20 admirably succeeds in advising us how to do the best job that can be done at this point to diagnose, understand, measure, and treat some of the most challenging conditions that prompt patients to seek psychiatric help.

Foreword

Katharine A. Phillips, M.D.

The somatoform and factitious disorders are fascinating syndromes that are beset with contradictions. They have an unusually long, rich, and colorful historical and clinical tradition, yet some of them have received scant empirical investigation. Most of the somatoform disorders appear to be relatively common in a diverse array of clinical settings—psychiatric, primary care, and specialty medical settings—yet they often go unrecognized and undiagnosed. In addition, although the somatoform disorders are grouped together in a separate diagnostic section of DSM-IV-TR, they are unlikely to be closely related.

The somatoform disorders—somatization disorder, undifferentiated somatoform disorder, conversion disorder, pain disorder, hypochondriasis, and body dysmorphic disorder (BDD)—involve a focus on bodily/somatic complaints. A general medical condition, substance use, or another mental disorder does not fully account for the physical symptoms or concerns, and the physical symptoms are not intentionally produced (unlike factitious disorders). Although it is often said that the common feature of these disorders is the presence of physical symptoms that suggest a general medical condition, this is not the case for BDD, which instead consists of a preoccupation with a perceived appearance flaw. Factitious disorders are characterized by physical or psychological symptoms, which, unlike the somatoform disorders, are intentionally produced or feigned by the patient in order to assume the sick role.

This book provides a clinically focused overview of these complex disorders. Undifferentiated somatoform disorder (a residual category for somatoform presentations that do not meet criteria for somatization disorder or another somatoform disorder) is not included. Pain disorder, which was included in *Review of Psychiatry*, Volume 19 (2000), is also excluded. Although factitious disorders are classified in a separate section of DSM-IV-TR, they are included here because they often consist of prominent somatic symptoms, and in clinical settings they can be difficult to differentiate from the somatoform disorders. Indeed, as discussed in Chapter 5, the somatoform disorders and factitious disorder may not be discrete and distinct, but may instead be on a continuum.

As the following chapters illustrate, most of the somatoform disorders appear to be relatively common in psychiatric and other medical settings, although further studies of their prevalence are needed. Some of these disorders present more often to primary care physicians, neurologists, internists, dermatologists, and surgeons than to psychiatrists. Psychiatrists nonetheless often see these patients, but because the presenting symptoms can be covert (as in the case of BDD, for example) or unusually complex (when attempting to differentiate seizures from pseudoseizures, for example), the somatoform disorders may go unrecognized or be diagnosed incorrectly. The factitious disorders appear to be more common in medical settings than is generally appreciated, and they are among the most memorable and difficult cases that clinicians encounter.

Most of the chapters in this book convey the unusually rich history of somatoform and factitious disorders. The intriguing symptoms with which patients present have captivated and vexed clinicians for millennia. The *Papyrus Ebers,* an Egyptian medical document that dates back to 1600 B.C., discussed "hysteria," a term previously used to describe somatoform symptoms. Hippocrates, who believed that a wandering uterus caused pain and disease in women, designed treatments such as body bandaging to restrict uterus movement. In medieval times, "major hysteria" was explained by demonic possession. Some of the most renowned physicians of recent centuries (e.g., Janet, Charcot, Freud) labored to solve the many mysteries of these disorders.

Despite the consistent richness of their historical and clinical tradition, somatoform and factitious disorders have received variable, and in some cases limited, empirical investigation. One exception is somatization disorder. For decades researchers have applied an unusually careful and systematic approach to developing and refining the diagnostic criteria for this disorder, and elegant family and adoption studies have been conducted. Research on hypochondriasis has delineated its phenomenology, comorbidity, and assessment, greatly advancing our understanding of the disorder. Although systematic research on BDD has only recently begun, our knowledge of this underrecognized disorder has rapidly increased during the past decade. Treatment of the somatoform and factitious disorders has received less empirical investigation than that of many other major mental illnesses; nonetheless, recent and ongoing research continues to increase knowledge of effective pharmacologic and psychotherapeutic treatment strategies for these distressing and impairing disorders.

One question addressed by several authors in this book is whether the somatoform disorders are actually related. DSM-IV-TR (p. 485) classifies these disorders on the basis of "clinical utility (i.e., the need to exclude occult general medical conditions or substance-induced etiologies for the bodily symptoms) rather than on assumptions regarding shared etiology or mechanism." This classification does have some clinical utility, and the disorders are similar in content (i.e., a focus on the body). However, they seem dissimilar in form and are likely to have distinct etiologies.

The form, or structure, of BDD and one form of hypochondriasis, for example, is characterized by prominent obsessions and compulsive behaviors, making it more similar to that of obsessive-compulsive disorder (OCD) than the other somatoform disorders. Complicating this picture, however, is that other forms of hypochondriasis appear to be more similar to depressive disorders or somatization disorder than to OCD. The form, or structure, of conversion disorder, in particular, differs considerably from that of BDD. Rather than involving prominent obsessions and repetitive behaviors, conversion disorder consists of symptoms or deficits affecting voluntary motor or sensory function, such as paralysis, aphonia, or diplopia. Although the mechanism by which conversion symptoms develop is not entirely clear, dissociation appears to play an important role. Indeed, it has been argued that conversion disorder shares essential phenomenologic features with the dissociative disorders and should be classified with them, as in ICD-10. On the other hand, conversion disorder also appears to be related to certain somatoform disorders, particularly somatization disorder and pain disorder.

The chapters that follow offer a broad and scholarly synthesis of much of the current knowledge, as well as current controversies, about somatoform and factitious disorders. They provide up-to-date, clinically focused overviews of these intriguing and often difficult to treat conditions, which practicing psychiatrists are likely to encounter regardless of the setting in which they work.

Chapter 1

Somatization Disorder

Vicenzio Holder-Perkins, M.D.
Thomas N. Wise, M.D.

Somatic symptoms may be conceptualized as warning individuals of potential dangers to their health and well-being, but these symptoms also have an interpersonal dimension that alerts the larger social environment to the need for relief from usual activities (Engel 1959). For example, mothers respond to what is perceived as somatic discomfort in their infants, which fosters a bond between the infant and parent that can evolve into a prototype as the infant matures. Using this developmental model, early psychoanalytic theorists considered basic unconscious mechanisms to explain physical symptoms as a compromise formation for basic unconscious conflict (primary gain) and avoidance of specific tasks (secondary gain). Thus, in early psychiatric approaches to somatization, unexplained medical symptoms were primarily derived from a theory that was difficult to test.

The term "somatization" is used differently by various authors. In reviewing both the term and the concept, Lipowski (1987) considered somatization to be a process as well as a disorder. He suggested that the most useful definition of somatization is from Kleinman (1982), in which somatization is defined as a "somatic idiom of psychosocial distress." In research studies, somatization has been operationalized in three ways: 1) as medically unexplained somatic symptoms, 2) as hypochondriacal worry or somatic preoccupation, and 3) as somatic clinical presentations of affective, anxiety, or other psychiatric disorders (Barsky et al.

The authors would like to acknowledge Darvin E. Williams and Suzanne Evans, who assisted in the production of this chapter.

1992a, 1992b; Goldberg and Bridges 1988; Janca et al. 1995; Kirmayer and Robbins 1991). In DSM-IV (American Psychiatric Association 1994), somatization disorder refers to a diagnostic entity with specific diagnostic criteria (Table 1–1). However, the term "somatization" is often imprecisely used to refer to the larger category of DSM-IV somatoform disorders. The somatoform disorder section in DSM-IV reflects disorders in which somatic complaints are central issues as opposed to merely unexplained physical symptoms or other applications of the concept of somatization. The somatoform disorders include not only somatization disorder, but also hypochondriasis, undifferentiated somatoform disorder, conversion disorder, pain disorder, and body dysmorphic disorder.

In this overview, somatization disorder refers to the DSM diagnosis, which is characterized by a lifetime history beginning before age 30 of seeking treatment for or becoming impaired by multiple physical complaints that cannot be fully explained by a general medical condition, or are in excess of what would be expected from examination, and are not intentionally feigned as seen in malingering or factitious disorders. However, where indicated, the broader concept of somatization as defined previously is also referred to.

Evolution of Diagnostic Criteria

The term "hysteria" has been used since Hippocrates. Hysteria is characterized by recurrent, multiple somatic complaints that are often described dramatically and are not explained by known clinical disorders. Hysteria was Freud's central concern during the early years of psychoanalysis, and ultimately resulted in the conceptualization of conversion as a defensive mechanism in patients with hysteria. The patients Freud treated for hysteria had loss of motor and sensory functions that were not explained anatomically.

The aim of the defense against the painful idea (repression), according to Freud, was to weaken the painful idea by divesting its affect through diversion of the energy of the affect into somatic channels; to denote this, Freud proposed the term "conversion"

Table 1–1. DSM-IV-TR criteria for somatization disorder

A. A history of many physical complaints beginning before age 30 years that occur over a period of several years and result in treatment being sought or significant impairment in social, occupational, or other important areas of functioning.

B. Each of the following criteria must have been met, with individual symptoms occurring at any time during the course of the disturbance:

    (1) *four pain symptoms:* a history of pain related to at least four different sites or functions (e.g., head, abdomen, back, joints, extremities, chest, rectum, during menstruation, during sexual intercourse, or during urination)

    (2) *two gastrointestinal symptoms:* a history of at least two gastrointestinal symptoms other than pain (e.g., nausea, bloating, vomiting other than during pregnancy, diarrhea, or intolerance of several different foods)

    (3) *one sexual symptom:* a history of at least one sexual or reproductive symptom other than pain (e.g., sexual indifference, erectile or ejaculatory dysfunction, irregular menses, excessive menstrual bleeding, vomiting throughout pregnancy)

    (4) *one pseudoneurological symptom:* a history of at least one symptom or deficit suggesting a neurological condition not limited to pain (conversion symptoms such as impaired coordination or balance, paralysis or localized weakness, difficulty swallowing or lump in throat, aphonia, urinary retention, hallucinations, loss of touch or pain sensation, double vision, blindness, deafness, seizures; dissociative symptoms such as amnesia; or loss of consciousness other than fainting)

C. Either (1) or (2):

    (1) after appropriate investigation, each of the symptoms in Criterion B cannot be fully explained by a known general medical condition or the direct effects of a substance (e.g., a drug of abuse, a medication)

    (2) when there is a related general medical condition, the physical complaints or resulting social or occupational impairment are in excess of what would be expected from the history, physical examination, or laboratory findings

D. The symptoms are not intentionally produced or feigned (as in factitious disorder or malingering).

Source. Reprinted with permission from American Psychiatric Association: *Diagnostic and Statistical Manual of Mental Disorders,* 4th Edition, Text Revision. Washington, DC, American Psychiatric Association, 2000, p. 490. Copyright 2000, American Psychiatric Association.

(Jones 1963). In the absence of specific diagnostic criteria and systematic studies, the terms "hysteria" and "conversion" during the early years of psychoanalysis were inconsistent and confusing. Many psychoanalysts consider hysteria a simulation of illness designed to work out unconscious conflicts. A classic case of hysteria in the psychoanalytic literature is referred to by Jones (1963).

> The patient was an unusually intelligent girl of twenty one, who developed a museum of symptoms in connection with her father's fatal illness. Among them were paralysis of three limbs with contractures and anesthesias, severe and complicated disturbances of sight and speech, inability to take food, and a distressing nervous cough.

"Conversion" has sometimes been used as a synonym for "hysteria." This has led to difficulties in demarcating somatization from similar phenomena. The term "somatization" was coined by Stekel (1943) to define a bodily disorder that arises as the expression of a deep-seated neurosis, especially a "disease of the conscious" (Hinsie and Campbell 1970). Steckel regarded somatization as identical to Freud's concept of conversion.

A systematic approach to the diagnosis of hysteria began in 1859 with the published monograph, Traite clinique et therapeutique a l'hysterie, by the French physician Pierre Briquet (Mai and Merskey 1980), who described a young woman with multiple somatic complaints. Savill, an English physician, provided a similar description (Savill 1909). The contemporary approach to somatization was initiated by Cohen et al. (1953) at Harvard and later by Guze (1983) and Guze et al. (1986). Purtell et al. (1951) observed that a small cohort of individuals accounted for a majority of unexplained medical complaints and absenteeism as a result of health problems in textile mills near Boston. These individuals were primarily young women who had always thought of themselves as "sickly" and who complained of a wide variety of physical problems. The investigators categorized this syndrome as hysteria, which they later called "Briquet's syndrome." Briquet's syndrome eventually became somatization disorder in DSM-III (American Psychiatric Association 1980) (Cloninger 1986).

The development of the syndrome of somatization disorder, initially called "Briquet's syndrome," allowed it to be demarcated from conversion hysteria. Somatization disorder is polysymptomatic, has a chronic course, and primarily affects women. It is characterized by multiple unexplained somatic complaints in various organ systems, with patients presenting in a dramatic manner. Conversion phenomena, in contrast, were thought to be best used to describe symptoms restricted to the neurologic system that had no clear physiologic basis. The criteria for the original diagnosis of Briquet's syndrome proposed by Perley and Guze (1962) required the presence of 25 of a possible 59 medically unexplained symptom complaints and 9 of 10 symptom groups. In subsequent iterations of somatization disorder, clinicians have used successively fewer complaints to make the diagnosis. In DSM-III, 37 potential symptoms were considered, and in DSM-III-R (American Psychiatric Association 1987), 35 possible symptoms were included in the criteria. The diagnostic concordance between DSM-III and the original Perley and Guze criteria was a kappa of 0.6 (Brown and Smith 1991). Nevertheless, it became apparent that it was difficult for clinicians to remember such a long list of somatic symptoms, and DSM-IV developed briefer diagnostic criteria that were both accurate and more usable in clinical settings. The DSM-IV criteria require a history of unexplained pain in at least four different sites, two gastrointestinal symptoms other than pain that have no clear organic explanation, an unexplained genitourinary or sexual symptom other than pain, and at least one medically unexplained symptom suggestive of a pseudoneurologic disorder that is not limited to pain (e.g., a conversion symptom or dissociation) (Table 1–1). These criteria demonstrated excellent concordance with the original Briquet's syndrome diagnostic criteria (kappa = 0.79, sensitivity = 81%, specificity = 96%) (Cloninger and Yutzy 1993).

However, there are several problems with the current definition of somatization disorder. These include the restrictive diagnostic criteria, the focus on symptom counting, and the failure to include aspects of this disorder such as behavior, cognitive attribution, and personality. In addition, the clinical status of individuals whose symptoms do not meet DSM-IV criteria for somatization disorder, but who are troubled by their medically unexplained complaints, is unclear. Several studies have suggested including an abridged or subsyndromal form of somatization in the official psychiatric nosology (DSM). Rief and Hiller (1999) proposed the term "polysymptomatic somatoform disorder" to refer to the presence of at least 7 unexplained physical symptoms affecting multiple body sites during the past 2 years. In addition to symptom counting, the authors included psychological factors associated with physical symptoms (e.g., sustained focused attention on bodily processes or a general tendency to misinterpret bodily sensations as evidence of physical illness). Escobar et al. (1989) also proposed a less severe form of somatization disorder. This form requires the presence of 4 or more physical symptoms for men and 6 or more symptoms for women of the 40 specific somatization symptoms included in the Composite International Diagnostic Interview. These symptoms must reach certain severity levels and be medically unexplained. There is no age-at-onset requirement for this syndrome. Swartz et al. (1986) also defined a subsyndromal form of somatization disorder associated with higher rates of health care–seeking behavior than in the general population but lower rates of health care–seeking behavior than in patients with DSM-defined somatization disorder; 11.6% of the general population met criteria for this category. Kroenke et al. (1997) also introduced a subsyndromal form of somatization disorder called "multisomatoform disorder." This concept stressed the presence of 3 or more current somatoform symptoms from a 15-symptom checklist along with at least a 2-year history of somatoform symptoms.

Ethnographic research by Kirmayer and Young (1998) urged the inclusion of cultural meanings of symptoms in the development of somatization classification criteria. These and other researchers proposed the potential utility of viewing somatization as a continuum on which increasing degrees of somatic symptoms indicate increasing distress, disability, and maladaptive illness behavior (Lipowski 1987). The clinical utility of this broader concept is significant in that it may better identify treatable somatizing patients with comorbid psychiatric disorders (anxiety or depression) in primary care settings (Lipowski 1990).

Epidemiology

Somatization as a behavior is common in all cultures and thus may not constitute a medical or psychiatric disorder. Population-based surveys have shown that 85%–95% of community respondents experienced at least one physical symptom every 2–4 weeks (White et al. 1961). Demers et al. (1980) found that patients presenting to primary care physicians noted a new symptom in a health care diary every 5–7 days, few of which were brought to a physician's attention and even fewer of which received a diagnosis.

In the general population, somatization disorder (as defined by DSM-III) is quite rare. In the Epidemiologic Catchment Area (ECA) study, somatization disorder was found in 0.01% of the population (Robins and Regier 1991). Individuals with somatization disorder are generally found in the general medical sector and rarely seek psychiatric care unless urged to do so by their primary care physicians (Smith et al. 1986). However, in other population samples (e.g., primary care), the abridged or subsyndromal form of somatization has been found to be common. In a community sample ($n = 3,132$), using slightly varying definitions, Escobar et al. (1987) reported a rate of subsyndromal somatization disorder of 4.4%–20.0% compared with only 0.3%–0.7% for the full DSM-III somatization disorder diagnosis. Kroenke et al. (1997), in a study of 1,000 primary care patients, reported that 8% met criteria for "multisomatoform disorder." Using the Swartz et al. (1986) abridged definition of somatization disorder, a prevalence of 11.6% was found in the general population $n = 3,793$). A large international study conducted in 15 primary care centers ($n = 5,438$) in 14 countries found that the prevalence of ICD-10 (World Health Organization 1992) somatization disorder was 2.8%, whereas the prevalence of abridged somatization as measured by the Somatic Symptom Index was 19.7% (Gureje et al. 1997).

Researchers have investigated other epidemiologic aspects of somatization, such as gender, socioeconomic status, educational level, and immigrant status. Females somatize more than males, and individuals of lower socioeconomic status somatize more than those of higher socioeconomic status (Wool and Barsky 1994). In the ECA study, somatization disorder was most prevalent among

African American women (0.8%), followed by African American men (0.4%) (Robins and Regier 1991). These findings may be accounted for by educational status. Somatization disorder was no more prevalent among Hispanic Americans than other groups. However, in the Puerto Rican ECA study ($n = 1,513$), the rate of somatization disorder was 10 times higher than in the United States population, even after taking sociodemographic variables, including educational level, into account (Escobar 1987). Ritsner et al. (2000) conducted a study to examine the prevalence of somatization in an immigrant population in Israel ($n = 966$) and reported a 6-month prevalence rate of 21.9%.

Clinical Features

Somatization disorder consists of multiple recurrent physical symptoms and complaints in multiple organ systems that cannot be objectively validated (e.g., by physical examinations or diagnostic studies) or cannot be fully explained on the basis of a known medical condition or the direct effect of a substance. These unexplained physical complaints must begin before age 30 and assume a chronic and fluctuating course. They must consist of at least four pain symptoms, two gastrointestinal symptoms, one sexual symptom, and one pseudoneurologic symptom. In addition, the physical symptoms and complaints are usually of sufficient severity to impair social, occupational, or other important areas of functioning (Table 1–1).

Patients with somatization disorder may present with a history of a large number of outpatient visits, frequent hospitalization, and repetitive subspecialty referrals. It is imperative that medical history not be overlooked, because the diagnosis can be missed. The medical record may reveal the use of multiple medications and a large number of diagnoses and diagnostic studies. This is a concrete manifestation of the somatically preoccupied patient's high utilization of health care resources. Patients with somatization disorder have been found to have a threefold higher use of ambulatory services, a 50% higher use of office visits, and a ninefold higher overall cost for health care than nonsomatically preoccupied patients in the United States (Hollifield et al. 1999).

Etiologic Considerations

Defense Mechanism/Conflict Resolution

Psychodynamic theorists have traditionally conceptualized somatization as a neurosis, an unconscious process that leads to a maladaptive use of defense mechanisms, which could give rise to a bodily disorder. The literature is replete with case histories, and clinical experience suggests that some individuals use bodily metaphors as an expression of emotional distress. However, this concept is complex and difficult to test empirically, which likely explains the paucity of empirical studies. This does not preclude the possibility that these mechanisms play a substantial role in somatization disorder, at least in some individuals.

Genetic/Family Studies

There is an increased rate of somatization disorder in first-degree female relatives of patients with somatization disorder, indicating familial aggregation of the disorder (Guze and Cloninger 1986). Family studies have linked somatization disorder to antisocial personality disorder (Cloninger et al. 1975; Coryell 1980); first-degree male relatives of patients with somatization disorder have elevated rates of both antisocial personality and alcoholism. Cloninger et al. (1975) used an alternative method to assess the association between antisocial personality disorder and somatization disorder: by examining first-degree relatives of male felons. This study found an increased rate of somatization disorder in female relatives. The investigators suggested that sociopathy and somatization may have a common etiology. Further strengthening these findings, a study of adopted children whose biologic parents had antisocial behaviors revealed a higher-than-expected rate of hysteria or other multiple unexplained somatic complaints in female offspring (Cadoret et al. 1976; Sandler et al. 1984; Wessely 1999).

Behavior/Learning Theories

Several theories have proposed that somatization results from social learning or modeling of illness behavior and that childhood exposure to models of illness behavior, such as an ill parent, may increase the risk for somatization. Craig et al. (1993) and Bass and Murphy (1995) found that a high percentage of patients with somatization disorder had parents who were physically ill. Jamison and Walker (1992) observed that children of adults with chronic pain reported more abdominal pain and used more analgesics than a normative control group. The consequences of another's behavior may inhibit or reinforce a child's behavior by signifying which patterns of illness behavior are appropriate and likely to be reinforced, and which are socially unacceptable and likely to be punished (Craig 1978).

Early Life Experiences

Other early life experiences proposed to explain somatizing behavior include childhood illness and childhood trauma. Craig et al. (1993) found that adults with a variety of somatoform disorders reported more frequent and serious childhood illnesses than other psychiatric and medical patients. There is also evidence that parental responses to childhood illness and inadequate or inattentive parenting may contribute to somatizing illnesses. Stuart and Noyes (1999) reviewed research on childhood antecedents and personality contributions to somatoform disorders. They hypothesized that somatizing behavior may be best understood as a unique form of interpersonal behavior that is driven by anxious and maladaptive attachment styles. This pattern promotes more intense care-seeking behavior and is self-defeating in that it may ultimately lead to rejection by others, further fueling the treatment-seeking behavior.

Physical and sexual abuse have also been linked to somatization disorder. Walling et al. (1994) observed that childhood physical abuse was a better predictor of somatization disorder than other early traumatic experiences. Morrison (1989) reported that 55% of women with somatization disorder, compared with 16% of women with affective disorders, reported a history of sexual abuse. Regarding somatizing behavior more broadly, chronic pelvic pain and abdominal functional symptoms are more common in women who were sexually abused in childhood (Leserman et al. 1998; Walker et al. 1996). Other studies have extended the focus from gynecologic to gastrointestinal symptoms, because they are related to organ systems that are targets of abuse. Reilly et al. (1999) studied male and female adult patients with nonepileptic seizures or irritable bowel syndrome and compared them with a similar group of patients with epilepsy and Crohn's disease. The authors concluded that adults presenting with functional neurologic and abdominal symptoms had an increased recollection of sexual and physical abuse, as both children and adults.

Personality

As previously noted, earlier family studies proposed a link between antisocial personality disorder and somatization disorder or Briquet's syndrome (Cloninger et al. 1975; Coryell 1980; Guze and Cloninger 1986). However, more recent studies did not find any specific personality disorder to be more common among patients with somatization disorder (Emerson et al. 1994; Rost et al. 1992; Stern et al. 1993). The most frequent personality disorders reported by Rost and colleagues in a group of somatizing patients referred from primary care settings were avoidant, paranoid, self-defeating, and obsessive-compulsive personality disorders. Antisocial personality disorder was observed in only 7% of the 61% of somatizing patients with an identified personality disorder.

Several studies have suggested that alexithymia may be associated with somatization disorder (Taylor et al. 1997). The term "alexithymia" means the inability to verbalize one's emotions. Sifneos (1973), who coined the term, observed that patients with psychosomatic disorders have difficulties expressing emotions verbally and do not have fantasies or feelings. In a Finnish study of primary health care patients in an urban setting, alexithymia was associated with frequent use of health care services (Joukamaa et al. 1996). Alexithymia correlates positively with depression, hypochondriasis, and somatization disorder as well as a tendency to report physical symptoms (Cohen et al. 1994; Kauhanen et al. 1991).

Differential Diagnosis

The differential diagnosis of unexplained medical complaints includes a number of psychiatric disorders (Table 1–2). Major depressive disorder can present with fatigue, dizziness, weight change, and other somatic complaints. The salient difference between somatization disorder and a depressive disorder is that the central feature of somatization disorder is medically unexplained somatic symptoms, whereas in depression the patient's depressed mood fosters a sense of helplessness and hopelessness concerning a variety of situations, not just health concerns. It is important to ascertain whether the patient has a life-long history of unexplained medical complaints, or whether physical complaints are limited to depressive episodes. Such a history often becomes apparent if the patient with somatization disorder had multiple hospitalizations and surgical procedures at a relatively early age for seemingly benign conditions.

Anxiety disorders, panic disorders in particular, may have a variety of symptoms indicative of hyperarousal, such as subjective cardiac palpitations, rapid breathing, and chest pain or tension, which may be misinterpreted as the onset of a myocardial infarction or an asthma attack. However, the symptoms of somatization disorder are not limited to the cardiopulmonary system; they involve multiple organ systems. In addition, unlike an individual with anxiety symptoms, fear and excessive worry are not central to somatization disorder. The anxiety sensitivity in the panic disorder patient consists of an internal scanning for the development of a panic attack rather than the presentation of multiple medically unexplained symptoms that do not resemble an acute anxiety attack. Exclusion of psychotic disorders (e.g., schizophrenia, delusional disorder) is essential when evaluating medically unexplained somatic symptoms. Psychotic disorders may have as a central theme a bizarre bodily delusion (e.g., that extraterrestrial beings are causing abdominal pain). In somatization disorder, the beliefs are not bizarre or of delusional intensity.

Conversion disorder is limited to symptoms that affect the voluntary motor or sensory functions of the neurologic system. In pain disorder, pain is the predominant focus of the clinical presentation, unlike in somatization disorder. Unlike patients with

Table 1–2. Differential diagnosis of somatization disorder

Disorder	Comments
Major depressive disorder	A disorder marked by depressed mood; inability to concentrate; disturbed appetite, libido, and sleep patterns; and diminished interest in usual activities. Somatic complaints occur in the context of these symptoms.
Panic disorder	A disorder marked by acute onset of anxiety, accompanied by autonomic arousal that abates. Concerns about disease, such as a heart attack, may follow, but are not a central focus.
Psychotic disorders	In psychotic disorders marked by delusions of disease, the delusion is intense and may be interpreted as being bizarre.
Conversion disorder	A disorder marked by sensory or voluntary motor deficit thought to be associated with psychological factors.
Pain disorder	A disorder in which pain is the primary focus of the complaint. Psychological factors are thought to play a role in the pain's severity and maintenance.
Hypochondriasis	A disorder in which the individual has a fearful preoccupation that he or she has a serious illness or in which the individual misinterprets bodily symptoms as indicating that he or she has a serious disease. Despite reassurance through medical evaluation and testing, the preoccupation continues.

somatization disorder, those with hypochondriasis are "explanation-seekers" rather than treatment seekers (Barsky et al. 1994; Starcevic et al. 1992).

Evaluating the Patient With Somatization Disorder

Somatization disorder, if not recognized by the clinician, may lead to frustration for the clinician and patient, mutual rejection by the clinician and patient, as well as unnecessary medical expenditures and risk of iatrogenic illness. It is a disorder that is often elusive; therefore, clinicians must have a high index of suspicion. At the first session, the clinician should carefully evaluate the patient based on an understanding of the evolution of the patient's illness and health-related experiences.

In the initial evaluation phase, the patient presents to the clinician with specific symptoms and signs to which the clinician responds with questions, physical examinations, laboratory tests, and radiographic studies. This process continues until the disorder is sufficiently organized to allow the clinician to diagnose the complaint syndromically. The process is disrupted if the clinician suggests to the somatizing patient that "it's all in your head." This negates the patient's subjective suffering, and the complaint will likely persist despite medical reassurance. The most significant undertaking for the clinician during this phase is to establish and maintain a good relationship with the patient. Quill (1985) wrote, "The most helpful intervention may be a caring, respectful long-term medical relationship not linked to testing, surgery or the resolution of symptoms."

Unfortunately, especially in primary care settings, there may be only a brief amount of time in which to gather data. Despite such limitations, it is essential that the clinician understand the meaning and context of symptoms for which there seem to be no organic etiology, yet persist and lead to illness and worry.

Brief questionnaires are available to clinicians to evaluate the patient's tendency to experience and report physical symptoms. These instruments are useful adjunctive measures for assessing patients with somatic preoccupations, although most do not diagnose somatization disorder per se (Table 1–3). The Primary Care Evaluation of Mental Disorders (PRIME-MD) (Spitzer et al. 1994) somatization subsection was developed to cover the 15 most common physical symptoms that patients present to primary care physicians (excluding respiratory symptoms). Three or more positive responses within the first 15 symptoms direct the primary care physician to the interview portion of the PRIME-MD for somatization disorder. A higher number of positive responses to these 15 PRIME-MD somatic symptoms correlates with an

Table 1–3.   Psychometric approaches to measuring somatization

Measure	Description
Primary Care Evaluation of Mental Disorders (PRIME-D)	Identifies mental disorders that are common in primary care. It consists of two components: a 1-page patient questionnaire (26 items) and a 12-page clinician evaluation guide or structured interview for follow-up on positive responses.
Whiteley Index	A 14-item "yes" or "no" questionnaire that screens for hypochondriasis. This measure distinguishes hypochondriacal from non-hypochondriacal patients.
Illness Behavioral Questionnaire	A 62-item inventory that assesses seven dimensions of general hypochondriasis, disease conviction, psychological versus somatic focus, affective inhibition, affective disturbance, denial, and irritability. The Whiteley Index of Hypochondriasis is derived from this scale.
Somatosensory Amplification Scale	A 10-item self-report inventory that measures an individual's sensitivity to bodily sensations that do not denote serious disease.
Health Attitude Survey	A 27-item questionnaire that assess somatization. It differs from other somatization screening instruments in that it avoids mention of physical symptoms and instead focuses on dissatisfaction with health and distress related to health problems.

increased risk of an anxiety or mood disorder and increased functional impairment.

The Whiteley Index screens for hypochondriasis and distinguishes hypochondriacal from nonhypochondriacal patients (Pilowsky 1978, 1987). The 62-item Illness Behavior Questionnaire (Pilowsky et al. 1979) has been widely used to examine dimensions of illness behavior such as denial, disease conviction, and hostility, whereas the Somatosensory Amplification Scale (Barsky and Wyshak 1990) quantifies how much an individual magnifies routine visceral sensations. All three questionnaires have been demonstrated to be valid and reliable in medical settings (Hollifield et al. 1999; Kellner 1991).

Noyes et al. (1999) designed the Health Attitude Survey to assess somatization. This 27-item scale differs from other somatization screening instruments in that it purposely avoids mention of physical symptoms. A number of items focus on psychological distress, somatic symptom presentation, health care utilization, interaction with physicians, and satisfaction with medical care. The survey showed acceptable predictive value and may prove useful in clinical settings in which rapid screening is desired.

The aforementioned questionnaires help the clinician further evaluate and discuss with patients their tendencies to amplify normal somatic sensations and their illness beliefs and fears. Use of these instruments can also facilitate communication with other clinicians.

Treatment Considerations

General Approach

Physicians often encounter difficulties in diagnosing and managing patients who are somatically preoccupied. A major issue is that these patients focus on somatic concerns and tend to deny psychological and social issues (Pilowsky 1978, 1987). The proclivity of somatization disorder to mimic medical conditions is another difficulty faced by the physician.

The general treatment of somatization disorder is based on data indicating that the disorder is chronic and that needless medical interventions and surgeries often accrue (Katon and Walker 1998). These data suggest that the most important element is conservative support and reassurance with minimal unnecessary interventions. Smith et al. (1986) documented that excess utilization of health care services could be reduced by one psychiatric consultation in which the primary care physician provides a clear referral note describing the disorder and explaining that such individuals tend to use a disproportionate amount of health care services and undergo unnecessary tests, procedures, and surgeries. This study was impressive in its efficient intervention and robust outcome. Direct attention to comorbid conditions, such as depression, anxiety, and substance abuse, is also essential. Treatment of the somatizing patient includes proper diagnosis, support, and reassurance (Smith et al. 1986).

Patients with somatization disorder may resist psychiatric intervention because such intervention may imply that "it's all in my head." The primary care physician should generally seek psychiatric consultation but not transfer the patient's care to the psychiatrist. It is important to note that psychiatric consultation is useful only when it is acceptable to the patient. The psychiatric consultation should provide a framework for treatment. Unwanted referrals to a psychiatrist might lead to feelings of rejection and fuel the patient's somatic complaints. Thus, if a referral is necessary, feelings of rejection should be discussed and the patient should be reassured that the primary care physician will continue to follow him or her. Because somatizing behavior may be fostered by real or perceived rejection responses from significant others, continued involvement and follow-up by the primary care physician is recommended (Smith 1988). The primary care physician should 1) schedule regular follow-up appointments of a set length; 2) set the agenda for the visits; 3) limit workups to objective findings, thus limiting iatrogenesis; 4) set limits on contacts outside clinical appointments; 5) explain that stress, both psychological and environmental, can cause physical symptoms; and 6) be careful about prescribing multiple medications to address unexplained symptoms in many organ systems (Smith 1988).

Psychotherapy

Various psychotherapies have been traditionally used to treat somatization disorder. Early clinical experience suggested that somatizing patients do not respond well to conventional insight-oriented psychotherapies (Ford 1983). Contemporary psychotherapies, such as time-limited cognitive behavioral therapy, appear more effective than open-ended psychoanalytically oriented strategies (Kellner 1986).

Cognitive-behavioral strategies are directed toward the cognitive, affective, and behavioral components of patients' symptoms. Clinicians should discuss with patients their tendency to employ catastrophic and negative thinking when they experience physiologic reactions and should illustrate the cognitions and behaviors that occur when patients experience unpleasant sensations. To help patients understand their affective responses to such sensations, the clinician can ask them to keep a behavioral log documenting their discomfort, the activities during which they experience discomfort, their emotional reactions, and the way they cope with the sensations. Essentially, patients and clinicians should pinpoint visceral sensations, the thoughts that were elicited by the discomfort, and the context in which the discomfort occurred. This allows a transition from a disease-focused worry to a broader understanding of the psychosocial context in which the discomfort occurred and facilitates identification of thoughts that automatically arose and the cognitive distortions that occurred. This cognitive approach may be done individually or in a group setting.

Primary care clinics at the Harvard Health Plan have established brief group therapy programs specifically for somatizing patients. Some of these programs have been remarkably effective in improving function and reducing distress. The sessions (8 to 16) combine general advice on topics such as stress management, problem solving, and social skills training, with specific interventions targeted at the mechanism of amplification and the need to be sick that underlies somatization. In a study of a 6-week group cognitive-behavioral intervention ($n = 171$), McLeod and Budd (1997) determined that patients experienced a decrease in emotional and physical distress, an increase in functional status, and a decrease in medical services utilization up to 12 months later. An inclusion criterion was unexplained somatic complaints, although not necessarily somatization disorder per se.

Reassurance is one of the most important modalities clinicians can use. Kathol (1997) suggests six steps that are needed to effectively reassure patients with benign disease or symptoms not explained by disease: 1) question and examine the patient, 2) assure the patient that serious illness is not present, 3) suggest that the symptom will resolve, 4) tell the patient to return to normal activity, 5) consider nonspecific treatment, and 6) follow the patient.

This approach acknowledges patients' suffering and their experiences of disability. Recognizing the somatic experience allows the clinician to take a more empathetic stance. In addition, the clinician's awareness of the behavioral reinforcers he or she controls may be helpful in changing unproductive patterns of interaction. Appropriate limits must be set, but the clinician must also make it clear that he or she is accessible to the patient, for it is this accessibility, rather than technical medical intervention, that is the mainstay of the treatment.

One way to help patients with an inability to deal with or communicate emotions (alexithymia) is to use nonverbal techniques, with the goal of helping the patient recognize the relationship between life situations and bodily reactions. Nonverbal therapies such as diet, meditation, physiotherapy, relaxation techniques, biofeedback, massage, and exercise are generally accepted by patients, as long as patients do not interpret their use as meaning that the physician is rejecting or discounting their somatic experience. Empirical evidence on the efficacy of these approaches is needed.

Psychotropic Medications

There is no medication available specifically for the treatment of somatization disorder. Nevertheless, patients with somatization disorder often seek medications from various physicians to treat each symptom. This may result in their taking large amounts of unnecessary medications. For this reason, it is best for only one physician, usually the primary care physician, to prescribe and manage all medications.

Psychotropic medications should be considered for comorbid psychiatric disorders, which are common in patients with somatization disorder (Lenze et al. 1999). However, it is imperative that the diagnosis of somatization disorder be established, because it may complicate treatment. Somatization disorder may potentiate drug-seeking behavior for comorbid disorders. Before prescribing benzodiazepines or narcotics, a thorough history of substance abuse or dependency should be explored and documented. The patient with an anxiety disorder, such as panic disorder, may require a benzodiazepine, and the postoperative patient may need opiates for pain management. In such situations, close monitoring of drug use is essential because patients with somatization disorder are at risk for abusing these medications. The use of selective serotonin reuptake inhibitors (SSRIs) or buspirone may be indicated to treat comorbid generalized anxiety disorder, and SSRIs and other newer antidepressant agents may be beneficial for comorbid depressive syndromes.

The somatizing patient is often sensitive to medication side effects; therefore, the physician should discuss in advance common side effects, explaining that these are normal responses to such medications. It is also important for the physician to inquire about other drugs, such as herbal preparations, that the patient may be taking, because drug interactions have the potential to cause adverse reactions.

Conclusion

Somatization disorder is a chronic and serious psychiatric disorder that frustrates patients, their families, and their physicians. Its chronic course and focus on somatic symptoms can lead to needless medical evaluations and potentially dangerous, unwarranted interventions. It is essential for physicians in all specialties to recognize this disorder and to understand its course, recognizing that the family matrix often includes alcoholism, antisocial personality, and similar somatization phenomena in a system that often does not recognize the psychological problems that challenge such patients. The treatment should consist of a conservative medical approach, with vigorous treatment of comorbid disorders such a depression or anxiety (Escobar et al. 1998). Subsyndromal somatization disorder is common in primary care settings and mandates similar therapeutic approaches. The psychiatrist can play an important role in the evaluation and diagnosis of such syndromes by educating physicians about this disorder and treating those patients who accept psychiatric treatment.

References

American Psychiatric Association: Diagnostic and Statistical Manual of Mental Disorders, 3rd Edition. Washington, DC, American Psychiatric Association, 1980

American Psychiatric Association: Diagnostic and Statistical Manual of Mental Disorders, 3rd Edition, Revised. Washington, DC, American Psychiatric Association, 1987

American Psychiatric Association: Diagnostic and Statistical Manual of Mental Disorders, 4th Edition. Washington, DC, American Psychiatric Association, 1994

American Psychiatric Association: Diagnostic and Statistical Manual of Mental Disorders, 4th Edition, Text Revision. Washington, DC, American Psychiatric Association, 2000

Barsky AJ, Wyshak G: Hypochondriasis and somatosensory amplification. Br J Psychiatry 157:404–409, 1990

Barsky AJ, Cleary PD, Wyshak G, et al: A structured diagnostic interview for hypochondriasis. A proposed criterion standard. J Nerv Ment Dis 180:20–27, 1992a

Barsky AJ, Wyshak G, Klerman GL: Psychiatric comorbidity in DSM-III-R hypochondriasis. Arch Gen Psychiatry 49:101–108, 1992b

Barsky AJ, Barnett MC, Cleary PD: Hypochondriasis and panic disorder: boundary and overlap. Arch Gen Psychiatry 51:918–925, 1994

Bass C, Murphy M: Somatoform and personality disorders: syndromal comorbidity and overlapping developmental pathways. J Psychosom Res 39:403–427, 1995

Brown FW, Smith GR Jr: Diagnostic concordance in primary care somatization disorder. Psychosomatics 32:191–195, 1991

Cadoret RJ, Cunningham L, Loftus R, et al: Studies of adoptees from psychiatrically disturbed biological parents. III. Medical symptoms and illnesses in childhood and adolescence. Am J Psychiatry 133: 1316–1318, 1976

Cloninger CR: Somatoform and dissociative disorders, in The Medical Basis of Psychiatry. Edited by Winokur G, Clayton PJ. Philadelphia, PA, WB Saunders, 1986, pp 123–151

Cloninger CR, Yutzy S: Somatoform and dissociative disorders: a summary of changes for DSM-IV, in Current Psychiatric Therapies. Edited by Dunner DL. Philadelphia, PA, WB Saunders, 1993, pp 310–314

Cloninger CR, Reich T, Guze SB: The multifactorial model of disease transmission: III. Familial relationship between sociopathy and hysteria (Briquet's syndrome). Br J Psychiatry 127:23–32, 1975

Cohen K, Auld F, Booker H: Is alexithymia related to psychosomatic disorder and somatizing? J Psychosom Res 38:119–127, 1994

Cohen ME, Robins E, Purtell JJ, et al: Excessive surgery in hysteria. JAMA 151:977–986, 1953

Coryell W: A blind family history study of Briquet's syndrome. Further validation of the diagnosis. Arch Gen Psychiatry 37:1266–1269, 1980

Craig KD: Social modeling influences of pain, in The Psychology of Pain. Edited by Sternbach RA. New York, Raven, 1978, pp 79–103

Craig TK, Boardman AP, Mills K, et al: The South London Somatisation Study. I: longitudinal course and the influence of early life experiences. Br J Psychiatry 163:579–588, 1993

Demers RY, Altamore R, Mustin H, et al: An explanation of the dimensions of illness behavior. J Fam Pract 11:1085–1094, 1980

Emerson J, Pankratz L, Joos S, et al: Personality disorders in problematic medical patients. Psychosomatics 35:469–473, 1994

Engel GL: "Psychogenic" pain and the pain-prone patient. Am J Med 26:899–911, 1959

Escobar JI: Cross-cultural aspects of the somatization trait. Hospital and Community Psychiatry 38:174–180, 1987

Escobar JI, Burnam MA, Karno M, et al: Somatization in the community. Arch Gen Psychiatry 44:713–718, 1987

Escobar JI, Manu P, Matthews D, et al: Medically unexplained physical symptoms, somatization disorder and abridged somatization: studies with the Diagnostic Interview Schedule. Psychiatric Developments 3:235–245, 1989

Escobar JI, Gara M, Waitzkin H, et al: DSM-IV hypochondriasis in primary care. Gen Hosp Psychiatry 20:155–159,1998

Ford CV: The Somatizing Disorders: Illness as a Way of Life. New York, Elsevier, 1983

Goldberg DP, Bridges K: Somatic presentations of psychiatric illness in primary care settings. J Psychosom Res 32:137–144, 1988

Gureje O, Simon GE, Ustun TB, et al: Somatization in cross-cultural perspective: a World Health Organization study in primary care. Am J Psychiatry 154:989–995, 1997

Guze SB: Studies in hysteria. Can J Psychiatry 28:434–437, 1983

Guze SB, Cloninger CR, Martin RL, et al: A follow up and family study of Briquet's syndrome. Br J Psychiatry 149:17–23, 1986

Hinsie LE, Campbell RJ: Psychiatric Dictionary, 4th Edition. New York, Oxford University Press, 1970, p 706

Hollifield M, Paine S, Tuttle L, et al: Hypochondriasis, somatization, and perceived health and utilization of health care services. Psychosomatics 40:380–386, 1999

Jamison RN, Walker LS: Illness behavior in children of chronic pain patients. Int J Psychiatry Med 22:329–342, 1992

Janca A, Burke JD, Isaac M: The World Health Organization somatoform disorders schedule. A preliminary report on design and reliability. Eur J Psychiatry 10:373–378, 1995

Jones E: The Life and Work of Sigmund Freud. New York, Anchor Books, 1963

Joukamaa M, Karlsson H, Sholman B, et al: Alexithymia and psychosocial distress among frequent attendance patients in health care. Psychother Psychosom 65:199–202, 1996

Kathol RG: Reassurance therapy: what to say to symptomatic patients with benign or non-existent medical disease. Int J Psychiatry Med 27:173–180, 1997

Katon WJ, Walker EA: Medically unexplained symptoms in primary care. J Clin Psychiatry 59(suppl 20):15–21, 1998

Kauhanen J, Julkunen J, Salonen JT: Alexithymia and perceived symptoms: criterion validity of the Toronto Alexithymia Scale. Psychother Psychosom 56:247–252, 1991

Kellner R: Somatization and Hypochondriasis. New York, Praeger-Greenwood, 1986

Kellner R: Psychosomatic Syndromes and Somatic Symptoms. Washington, DC, American Psychiatric Press, 1991

Kirmayer LJ, Robbins JM. Three forms of somatization in primary care: prevalence, co-occurrence, and sociodemographic characteristics. J Nerv Ment Dis 179:647–655, 1991

Kirmayer LJ, Young A: Culture and somatization: clinical, epidemiological, and ethnographic perspectives. Psychosom Med 60:420–430, 1998

Kleinman A: Neurasthenia and depression: a study of somatization and culture in China. Cult Med Psychiatry 6:117–190, 1982

Kroenke K, Spitzer RL, deGruy FV 3rd, et al: Multisomatoform disorder. An alternative to undifferentiated somatoform disorder for the somatizing patient in primary care. Arch Gen Psychiatry 54:352–358, 1997

Lenze EJ, Miller AR, Munir ZB, et al: Psychiatric symptoms endorsed by somatization disorder in a psychiatric clinic. Ann Clin Psychiatry 11:73–79, 1999

Leserman J, Li Z, Drossman DA, et al: Selected symptoms associated with sexual and physical abuse history among female patients with gastrointestinal disorders: the impact on subsequent health care visits. Psychol Med 28:417–425, 1998

Lipowski ZJ: Somatization: the experience and communication of psychological distress as somatic symptoms. Psychother Psychosom 47:160–167, 1987

Lipowski ZJ. Somatization and depression. Psychosomatics 31:13–21, 1990

Mai FM, Merskey H: Briquet's Treatise on Hysteria. A synopsis and commentary. Arch Gen Psychiatry 37:1401–1405, 1980

McLeod CC, Budd MA: Treatment of somatization in primary care: evaluation of the Personal Health Improvement Program. HMO Practice 11:88–94, 1997

Morrison J: Childhood molestation reported by women with somatization disorder. Ann Clin Psychiatry 1:25–32, 1989

Noyes R Jr, Langbehn DR, Happel RL, et al: Health Attitude Survey: a scale for assessing somatizing patients. Psychosomatics 40: 470–478, 1999

Perley MG, Guze SB: Hysteria: the stability and usefulness of clinical criteria. N Engl J Med 266:421–426, 1962

Pilowsky I: A general classification of abnormal illness behaviours. Br J Med Psychol 51:131–137, 1978

Pilowsky I: Abnormal illness behaviour. Psychiatr Med 5:85–91, 1987

Pilowsky I, Murrell TG, Gordon A: The development of a screening method for abnormal illness behaviour. J Psychosom Res 23:203–207, 1979

Purtell JJ, Robins E, Cohen ME: Observations on clinical aspects of hysteria. JAMA 146:902–909, 1951

Quill TE: Somatization disorder: one of medicine's blind spots. JAMA 254:3075–3079, 1985

Reilly J, Baker GA, Rhodes J, et al: The association of sexual and physical abuse with somatization: characteristics of patients presenting with irritable bowel syndrome and non-epileptic attack disorder. Psychol Med 29:399–406, 1999

Rief W, Hiller W: Toward empirically based criteria for the classification of somatoform disorders. J Psychosom Res 46:507–518, 1999

Ritsner M, Ponizovsky A, Kurs R, et al: Somatization in an immigrant population in Israel: a community survey of prevalence, risk factors, and help-seeking behavior. Am J Psychiatry 157:385–392, 2000

Robins LN, Regier D: Psychiatric Disorders in America: The Epidemiologic Catchment Area Study. New York, Free Press, 1991

Rost KM, Akins RN, Brown FW, et al: The comorbidity of DSM-III-R personality disorders in somatization disorder. Gen Hosp Psychiatry 14:322–326, 1992

Sandler RS, Drossman DA, Nathan HP, et al: Symptom complaints and health care seeking behavior in subjects with bowel dysfunction. Gastroenterology 87:314–318, 1984

Savill TD: Lectures on Hysteria and Allied Vasomotor Conditions. London, HJ Glaisher, 1909

Sifneos PE: The prevalence of alexithymic characteristics in psychosomatic patients. Psychother Psychosom 22:255–262, 1973

Smith GR Jr, Monson RA, Ray DC: Psychiatric consultation in somatization disorder. N Engl J Med 314:1407–1413, 1986

Smith RC: Somatization in primary care. Clin Obstet Gynecol 31:902–914, 1988

Spitzer RL, Williams JB, Kroenke K, et al: Utility of a new procedure for diagnosing mental disorders in primary care. The PRIME-MD 1000 study. JAMA 272:1749–1756, 1994

Starcevic V, Kellner R, Uhlenhuth EH, et al: Panic disorder and hypochondriacal fears and beliefs. J Affect Disord 24:73–85, 1992

Stekel W: The Interpretation of Dreams. New York, Liveright, 1943

Stern J, Murphy M, Bass C: Personality disorders in patients with somatisation disorder. A controlled study. Br J Psychiatry 163:785–789, 1993

Stuart S, Noyes R Jr: Attachment and interpersonal communication in somatization. Psychosomatics 40:34–43, 1999

Swartz M, Hughes D, George L, et al: Developing a screening index for community studies of somatization disorder. J Psychiatr Res 20:335–343, 1986

Taylor GJ, Bagby RM, Parker JDA: Disorders of Affect Regulation: Alexithymia in Medical and Psychiatric Illness. Cambridge, UK, Cambridge University Press, 1997

Walker EA, Gelfand AN, Gelfand MD, et al: Chronic pelvic pain and gynecological symptoms in women with irritable bowel syndrome. J Psychosom Obstet Gynaecol 17:39–46, 1996

Walling MK, O'Hara MW, Reiter RC, et al: Abuse history and chronic pain in women: II. A multivariate analysis of abuse and psychological morbidity. Obstet Gynecol 84:200–206, 1994

Wessely S: Functional somatic syndromes: one or many? Lancet 354:936–939, 1999

White K, Williams T, Greenberg B: The ecology of medical care. N Engl J Med 265:885–892, 1961

Wool CA, Barsky AJ: Do women somatize more than men? Gender differences in somatization. Psychosomatics 35:445–452, 1994

World Health Organization: International Statistical Classification of Diseases and Related Health Problems, 10th Revision. Geneva, World Health Organization, 1992

Chapter 2

Hypochondriasis

Brian A. Fallon, M.D.
Suzanne Feinstein, Ph.D.

The term "hypochondriasis" originated with the Greek belief that the source of emotional illness originated from the vapors emitted by the abdominal organs (below the ribs), causing a diffuse illness characterized primarily by either digestive symptoms (e.g., flatulence) or melancholia. In the late 17th century, Thomas Willis postulated that the brain was the source of both hypochondriasis in men and hysteria in women (Willis 1685) and added symptoms suggestive of panic disorder, such as trembling, palpitations, dizziness, and an imaginary fear of illness, to the description of hypochondriasis. In 1725, Sir Richard Blakemore, physician to the royal court of England, noted the legitimate suffering of patients with hypochondria and expressed remorse that they were so often treated with "derision and contempt." This physician may have been one of the first cognitive theorists in noting that "terrible ideas, formed only in the imagination, will affect the brain and the body with painful sensations" (Berrios 2001).

George Cheyne in 1733 elevated hypochondriasis to a disease of distinction, describing the disorder as "The English Malady," which afflicts persons of high intelligence and social class (Cheyne 1733). However, by the late 1800s, hypochondriasis had become considerably less fashionable and more pathological in that it was determined to be a disorder of brain function (Fabre 1847), which Savage (1892) described as causing "slight over-sensitiveness to insanity with marked delusions." Guislain (1852) categorized two types of hypochondria: melancholic or mental hypochondria and bodily hypochondria. In melancholic hypochondria, the patient felt physically weak, worried frequently about nonexistent diseases, and might have been preoccupied with suicidal thoughts. In bodily hypochondria, more frequently found in the community than in mental hospitals, the patient worried more about bodily symptoms than the disease implication itself. These descriptions were precursors to our current diagnoses of hypochondriasis, major depression with melancholic features, and somatization disorder. In today's nomenclature, hypochondriasis refers to a disorder in which there is an excessive fear or belief that one has a serious illness based on a misinterpretation of somatic symptoms; this fear or belief persists despite a physician's thorough examination and reassurance that a general medical disease is not present that could fully account for the patient's somatic concerns (American Psychiatric Association 1994). A patient with hypochondriasis may have a concomitant medical illness, but the degree of distress about illness far exceeds the seriousness of the symptoms themselves.

Clinical Features

Using the statistical tools of factor analysis, Pilowsky (1967) identified three key components of hypochondriasis: bodily preoccupation, disease phobia, and disease conviction. Depending on which feature is predominant in a particular patient, the disorder might appear strikingly different. For example, a patient with a high level of bodily preoccupation might check his or her body repeatedly or emphasize physical ailments when talking to others. A patient with a high level of disease phobia might avoid seeing a physician because he or she is terrified of hearing the physician confirm the fear: "Yes, you do have cancer." A patient with a high level of disease conviction may be the most difficult for a physician to tolerate, because such a patient responds with hostility to the physician's reassurance that no disease underlies the physical sensations. As the patient's mistrust and frustration rise, the physician in turn may come to resent the patient's anger, time demands, and disrespect of his or her medical authority (Barsky 1991). Such a strained doctor-patient relationship raises the risk that the patient with hypochondriasis may get a poor medical evaluation when in fact he or she may have a legitimate undetected physical illness.

The most common age at onset of hypochondriasis is in early adulthood, although it may occur at any age (Fallon et al. 1993). The course of hypochondriasis without treatment is thought to be chronic for the majority of patients, with symptoms waxing and waning in severity. With treatment, patients can do very well both in the short and long term. In a 4-year follow-up study (Barsky et al. 2000), patients with poor outcome tended to have a higher baseline tendency to amplify benign bodily sensations and attribute ambiguous sensations to bodily disease.

When the course is chronic, hypochondriasis may appear similar to lifetime obsessive-compulsive disorder (OCD) or a personality disorder. When the course is intermittent (Barsky et al. 1990) or of new onset, the physician should search for predisposing stressful life events as the cause (e.g., the sudden death of a loved one). Henry Maudsley, the great British anatomist of the 19th century, referred to this type of grief-induced hypochondria in poetic terms: "The sorrow that has no vent in tears makes other organs weep."

Patients with hypochondriasis frequently perform repetitive checking behaviors, such as asking family members and health care practitioners for reassurance, scheduling multiple doctor visits, and consulting medical books, to alleviate some of the anxiety caused by the somatic obsessions. In addition, many have a tendency to compulsively scan their bodies for signs of disease. Excessive probing and checking often aggravate the affected area and leave behind deceptive lumps and bumps, causing the patient and the physician to suspect the existence of disease. With the advent of the Internet, checking rituals may now include scanning medical Web sites for the signs and symptoms of illness and communicating online with other individuals who are experiencing anxiety. The Internet chat rooms can be particularly troubling sources of misinformation, leading one journalist who wrote about hypochondriasis to use the term "cyberchondria" (Carrns 1999).

An individual's degree of insight into the excessiveness of his or her fear of illness ranges from excellent to poor. For diagnostic purposes, patients with hypochondriasis who have little awareness of the unreasonable nature of their concerns should be diagnosed as having "hypochondriasis, with poor insight" (American Psychiatric Association 1994). Declining insight may lead to "overvalued ideation," which in turn may develop into hypochondriacal convictions of delusional intensity. If there is no insight at all into the possibility that the fear may be unfounded, and this lack of insight is sustained for long periods, patients should be diagnosed as having delusional disorder or major depression with psychotic features, not hypochondriasis.

The differential diagnosis of hypochondriasis is important to keep in mind when evaluating the patient. First, a medical condition must be excluded. Given that some medical diseases may be hard to exclude completely because their early stages are less apparent or because adequate laboratory diagnostic tools are unavailable for them (e.g., multiple sclerosis, systemic lupus erythematosus, Lyme disease, occult malignancies), the physician working with a patient whose hypochondriasis does not improve with psychiatric treatment should reconsider the possibility that a diagnosis of medical illness has been missed. Similar to somatization disorder, hypochondriasis is characterized by the presence of unexplained symptoms or sensations. However, the patient with hypochondriasis takes these symptoms one step further by leaping to a catastrophic cognitive misinterpretation of the significance of these symptoms.

One group of patients with hypochondriasis appears to have much in common with patients who have OCD (Barsky 1992; Fallon et al. 1991, 2000), particularly the intrusive obsessions about illness and the compulsive urges to check for reassurance. Patients with this OCD-like subtype of hypochondriasis are plagued by a heightened expectation of harm in the form of illness and pathological doubt over whether they were thorough enough in explaining their symptoms. The obsessional form of hypochondriasis needs to be considered when a patient asks a question such as "But doctor, how can I be sure?" This distinct subtype of hypochondria may have important therapeutic ramifications, because some medications particularly helpful for patients with OCD may also be helpful for patients with hypochondriasis.

Bienvenu et al. (2000) confirmed a relationship between OCD and hypochondriasis by demonstrating a higher frequency of hypochondriasis in patients with OCD and their first-degree family members than in control subjects and their first-degree family members.

Another group of patients with hypochondriasis appears to have symptoms of depression (Kellner et al. 1986b). The degree of insight of these patients tends to wax and wane less than that of patients with the obsessional form of hypochondriasis, and these patients have a more intense conviction that the illness is actually destroying them from within. Typically, these patients are tearful and suffer from concomitant major depression that emerged after the onset of hypochondriasis.

Theoretical Models

Psychodynamic Model

Psychodynamic understanding can contribute significantly to the therapist's ability to empathize with and treat patients with hypochondriasis. Further, an understanding of defense mechanisms can enhance treatment, perhaps allowing a therapeutic intervention from another theoretical school to be accepted, such as pharmacologic or cognitive-behavioral approaches.

Freud (1923/1961) postulated that the ego "is first and foremost a body ego." This concept led to the understanding that stress may precipitate regression, to the point that patients might report somatic symptoms rather than emotional turmoil. Freud (1914/1955) speculated that hypochondriasis stems from a turning inward of libidinal energy from external objects onto organs of the body, creating a bodily tension that demands the patient's full attention. Because this bodily tension may be experienced as both pleasurable and unpleasurable, the patient with hypochondriasis may be reluctant to relinquish symptoms.

Subsequent analytic theory has elaborated more comprehensive views of hypochondriasis. In one view, symptoms of hypochondriasis emerge as a compromise formation to protect the individual from overwhelming fears of punishment, bodily damage, and death that would be retaliation for the individual's sexual and aggressive feelings (Lipsitt 2001). Guilt over these feelings or impulses leads to fears of serious disease, preoccupation with bodily functions, a cycle of unpleasure and pleasure in interpersonal interactions, and dependency on others.

> Ms. D, a 45-year-old single woman with health fears and agoraphobia, was referred for treatment. Her history is notable for gastrointestinal distress, numerous negative medical workups, fears about serious illness secondary to the gastrointestinal complaints, and secondary panic attacks, which led to agoraphobia. Ms. D's physical complaints emerged shortly after her mother was hospitalized for a chronic debilitating medical disorder. Long the caregiver of her mother and one who had subverted many of her own passions and interests to her mother's needs, Ms. D found that she was no longer able to help her mother, or even to visit her mother, because of her own physical problems, illness preoccupation, and agoraphobia. Puzzled by her own deterioration and a near inability to leave her own home, Ms. D sought treatment. Within the first 10 sessions, it became apparent that Ms. D's relationship with her mother was a difficult one as a result of her mother's lifelong narcissism and psychological abuse. The therapeutic formulation was that Ms. D's desire to help was coupled with a repressed desire to harm her mother, an unconscious conflict that created extraordinary guilt and led to somatic punishment consisting of physical symptoms and hypochondriacal fears. After a session in which Ms. D proclaimed for the first time "I hate that woman's guts," she returned the following week with a smile, pronouncing that she was now able to leave her house and that her physical condition and illness fears had completely resolved. Over the subsequent months, her psychological state continued to improve remarkably. When her mother died, Ms. D felt further liberated and developed romantic interests for the first time in her life.

Although a psychodynamic understanding is a valuable component of any therapist-client interaction, psychodynamic psychotherapy may not be the most effective treatment for the majority of patients with hypochondriasis. In a prospective study of psychoanalytic psychotherapy for a series of patients with hypochondriasis who were chosen because they were believed to be good candidates for this intervention, Ladee (1966) found that only 4 (17%) of 23 patients experienced improvement at the end of treatment. Even though this is far from encouraging, significant advances have occurred both in the diagnosis of hypochondriasis and in the techniques of psychodynamic psychotherapy since the 1960s. Studies using standardized diagnostic methods, evaluation instruments, and treatment approaches will help determine the effectiveness of psychodynamic psychotherapy for patients with hypochondriasis.

Cognitive-Behavioral Model

Cognitive theorists have observed that excessive preoccupation with health is associated with negative and distorted thought patterns. In the cognitive formulation, hypochondriasis stems from faulty perceptions and unrealistic threat appraisals in which individuals misinterpret harmless bodily symptoms as having serious health implications. The perception of threat activates a "better safe than sorry" strategy, which was largely substantiated by Smeets et al. (2000), who found that patients with hypochondriasis adopted this strategy when faced with a health threat. This negative and distorted thought pattern causes patients to misinterpret medical communications, somatic symptoms, and changes in bodily functions as posing much greater threats than are realistic. Through selective memory and appraisal, patients filter medical information and physical changes that confirm an illness diagnosis while excluding incompatible information (Salkovskis 1996). As patients become increasingly hypervigilant about physical sensations that confirm an illness diagnosis, their misinterpretation of symptoms feeds the anxiety, often resulting in added physiological symptoms. Panic-type symptoms, such as increased sweating, acceleration of heart rate, dizziness, and shortness of breath, cause patients to become even further grounded in their beliefs that they have a serious illness (Salkovskis and Clark 1993). Subsequently, they perceive themselves to be helpless victims of their illness. The essence of cognitive therapy for hypochondriasis involves the identification and correction of this flawed belief system.

Because patients with hypochondriasis often have waxing and waning insight into the irrationality of their concerns, a psychological approach to the treatment of hypochondriasis may be more difficult when the patient is in the throes of low insight. Based on clinical experience, some cognitive therapists recommend structuring therapeutic interventions according to the degree of insight, using maximal training at times of higher insight, with the expectation that the principles learned will lead to less prolonged and less intense periods of low insight (Sisti 1997). Systematic investigation will help determine the impact of insight on therapeutic response.

A common characteristic of patients with the obsessional form of hypochondriasis is the manner in which they introduce uncertainty into the appraisal of situations most people would consider nonthreatening. Although there is no evidence of any health danger, these patients manifest continual doubt and attach uncertainty to circumstances that are potentially unsafe. For instance, patients often attach the possibility of harm to innocuous physiological changes or bodily sensations, ultimately activating the self-perpetuating obsessive cycle. One of the main attributes of this form of hypochondriasis is the need of patients to be reassured 100% that they do not have an illness. To compensate for this heightened uncertainty of a missed diagnosis, these patients impose excessive structure on their lives as well as inflexible limits and time markers. Thus, patients' inability to separate harmless aches and pains from more serious health threats results in either hypervigilance to bodily sensations, reassurance seeking as exhibited by excessive doctor visits, or avoidance behaviors. By identifying the irrationality of these thoughts, cognitive-behavioral therapists can help patients reattribute their false beliefs about their physical symptoms and health concerns (Warwick and Salkovskis 1989). Typical dysfunctional thoughts include the following (Salkovskis 1996, p. 66): "Bodily changes are usually a sign of serious disease, because every symptom has to have an identifiable physical cause." "If you don't go to the doctor as soon as you notice anything unusual then it will be too late." "If I don't worry about my health then I could get sick."

Patients with hypochondriasis resemble people with OCD in that they experience intrusive recurrent thoughts (in this case, obsessions about possible illness) and subsequently use covert and overt rituals to cope with stressors and reduce immediate discomfort. Sometimes people opt to use passive ritualistic behaviors (avoidance compulsions), such as circumventing doctor appointments and avoiding hospitals and sources of medical information, to counter or minimize the anxiety and discomfort caused by these thoughts. Dollard and Miller (1950) stated that avoidance tactics are usually unsuccessful in reducing anxiety related to obsessions because obsessions are frequently involuntary. Hence, active ritualistic behaviors are developed to counter the intrusive obsessions about illness.

Numerous controlled and uncontrolled studies suggest that cognitive and behavioral strategies can be helpful for patients with hypochondriasis (Table 2–1). Discussion of selected studies with larger samples sizes and formalized outcome measures follows.

In an uncontrolled retrospective study, Warwick and Marks (1988) found that 15 (88%) of 17 patients with hypochondriasis experienced significant improvement after seven sessions involving exposure and response prevention. Forty-six percent maintained improvement at 5-year follow-up. Therapists rated each patient's level of disability at home, at work, and during leisure time using a 9-point (0–8) scale. The exposure and response-prevention exercises were specifically tailored to the individual's health concerns. Examples of exposure exercises were visiting hospitals, reading relevant medical literature, repeatedly writing fears on paper, and deliberately inducing symptoms people associate with a heart attack through rigorous physical activity. Response-prevention exercises included deterring patients from seeking reassurance and preventing them from consulting medical books.

Warwick et al. (1996) randomized 32 patients with hypochondriasis to either a cognitive-behavioral therapy group or a no-treatment waiting-list control group. The cognitive-behavioral therapy group received weekly individual sessions of cognitive-behavioral therapy over a period of 4 months. After 4 months, the waiting-list control group received the same treatment. Evaluations were performed on both groups before randomization, and again at posttreatment/waiting-list control group stages. Further assessments were done at 3-month follow-up for the cognitive-

Table 2–1. Psychotherapeutic trials for treatment of hypochondriasis

Study	N	Design	Evaluation tools	Type of patient	Type(s) of therapy	Results	Comments
Kenyon 1964	118	Retrospective	Clinical interview	Inpatients	11% received supportive psychotherapy, 8% ECT	21% of all patients experienced improvement at discharge, 41% of all patients experienced improvement at 6-month follow-up	23% had comorbid affective or organic disorder
Ladee 1966	23	Prospective, noncontrolled	Clinical judgment	Outpatients	Psychoanalytic psychotherapy	17% experienced improvement	Patients were selected because they were believed to be good candidates for psychoanalytic psychotherapy
Goldstein and Birnbom 1976	4	Retrospective	Clinical interview	Geriatric outpatients	Psychotherapy	100% recovered	
Kellner 1983	45	Prospective	DSM-III clinical interview	Outpatients	Psychotherapy	64% experienced improvement or recovered	Improvement associated with absence of Axis II disorder and shorter illness duration
Warwick and Marks 1988	17	Retrospective	ICD-9 Fear Questionnaire, 9-point scale	Outpatients with DSM-III-R hypochondriasis	Exposure and response prevention	88% experienced significant improvement, 46% maintained improvement at 5-year follow-up	Comorbidity unknown, 59% dreaded future illness

Table 2–1. Psychotherapeutic trials for treatment of hypochondriasis (*continued*)

Study	N	Design	Evaluation tools	Type of patient	Type(s) of therapy	Results	Comments
Miller et al. 1988	7	Prospective	BDI, Spielberg Anxiety Illness Scale	Outpatients with DSM-III-R hypochondriasis	CBT	100% experienced improvement after 10 sessions, 86% maintained improvement at 3-month follow-up	
Stern and Fernandez 1991	6	Prospective	Hospital Anxiety and Depression Scale	Outpatients with DSM-III-R hypochondriasis	Group CBT	Significant decrease in number of physician visits	No change in amount of time spent worrying about illness
Logsdail et al. 1991	7	Retrospective	9-point scale	Nondepressed outpatients with DSM-III-R hypochondriasis	Exposure and response prevention	86% experienced significant improvement	57% diagnosed with hypochondriasis, 43% with OCD
Visser and Bouman 1992	6	Prospective crossover	BDI, IAS, MOCI, SCL-90	Outpatients with DSM-III-R hypochondriasis	Cognitive therapy and behavioral therapy	66% experienced significant improvement	Behavioral therapy appeared to be more effective than cognitive therapy
Warwick et al. 1996	32	Prospective	BAI, BDI, Visual Analog Scale	Outpatients with DSM-III-R hypochondriasis	CBT	76% experienced improvement after 16 sessions, improvement maintained at 3-month follow-up	

Table 2–1. Psychotherapeutic trials for treatment of hypochondriasis (*continued*)

Study	N	Design	Evaluation tools	Type of patient	Type(s) of therapy	Results	Comments
Bouman and Visser 1998	17	Prospective	BDI, IAS, MOCI, SCL-90	Outpatients with DSM-IV hypo-chondriasis	"Pure" cognitive or "pure" behav-ioral therapy	Patients in both groups experienced improvement	No significant differ-ences in effectiveness of cognitive therapy and behavioral therapy
Clark et al. 1998	48	Prospective	BAI, BDI, HARS, Visual Analog Scale, 18-item cognitive questionnaire	Outpatients with DSM-III-R hypo-chondriasis	Cognitive therapy, behavioral stress management therapy, or no-treatment waiting list	Both treatments were effec-tive at 1-year follow-up	Cognitive therapy was more effective than behavioral stress management therapy at 3 months
Fava et al. 2000	20	Prospective, random assignment	Self-report and observer-rated instruments, including CID and IAS	Outpatients with DSM-IV hypo-chondriasis	Explanatory therapy or no-treatment waiting list	Explanatory therapy resulted in significantly less severe hypochondriasis sustained over 6 months	Improvement noted, but substantial resid-ual symptoms remained

Note. BAI = Beck Anxiety Inventory; BDI = Beck Depression Inventory; CBT = cognitive-behavioral therapy; CID = Clinical Interview for Depression; ECT = electroconvulsive therapy; HARS = Hamilton Anxiety Rating Scale; IAS = Illness Attitude Scale; MOCI = Maudsley Obsessive-Convulsive Inventory; OCD = obsessive-compulsive disorder; SCL-90 = Symptom Checklist-90.

behavioral therapy group. After 16 sessions of cognitive-behavioral therapy, the cognitive-behavioral therapy group demonstrated significantly more improvement in hypochondriacal symptoms than the waiting-list control group and maintained improvement at 3-month follow-up. Despite certain study limitations, such as lack of reliability ratings as a result of using only one therapist and the fact that the waiting-list design did not control for the effects of attention, this study suggests that cognitive-behavioral therapy is effective for the treatment of hypochondriasis.

Bouman and Visser (1998) studied 17 patients with hypochondriasis before and after twelve 1-hour sessions with either "pure" cognitive therapy or "pure" behavioral therapy (exposure and response prevention). The cognitive therapy consisted of Beckian techniques (Beck and Emery 1985), in which therapists explained to patients that their irrational thoughts and exaggerated fears were the predecessors of their anxiety and distress. The cognitive therapists encouraged the patients to challenge their automatic thoughts to reduce their emotional and physical discomfort. Through identification of irrational thoughts, diaries, and subsequent cognitive restructuring, patients were able to successfully achieve reduction in hypochondriasis symptoms. Techniques used in the behavioral therapy consisted of prolonged and repeated exposure to moderately anxiety-provoking stressors to allow patients to habituate to their fears, ultimately leading to a reduction in anxiety. The behavior therapists created hierarchies of illness anxiety to help formulate a treatment plan. Patients were expected to complete homework assignments between weekly sessions in which they engaged in hierarchy-based exposure and response-prevention exercises. They also kept daily records of their illness anxieties and avoidance behaviors. When the behavior therapists compared specific measures of hypochondriasis (using the Illness Attitude Scale [Kellner 1987]) and depression before, during, and after treatment, patients demonstrated the most improvement during the active phase of treatment. During the 4-week no-intervention periods before and after treatment, patients did not show any changes in symptomatology. Results showed no significant differences in the effectiveness of cognitive therapy and behavioral therapy for treating hypochondriasis. Further investigation will reveal more about potentially confounding factors, such as therapist devotion, patient expectations for treatment, and patient-therapist rapport.

In a well-designed treatment study of hypochondriasis, Clark et al. (1998) improved on previous studies by employing several therapists for cognitive-behavioral treatment and randomly assigning 48 patients to behavioral stress management therapy, cognitive therapy, or a waiting-list control group. The behavioral stress management therapy consisted of applied relaxation training, detailed education about alternative explanations for symptoms, and behavioral techniques to reduce worrying time. Patients in the waiting-list control group were later randomized to either behavioral stress management therapy or cognitive therapy, with both treatments matched in terms of structured homework assignments, therapist time, patients' assessment of treatment legitimacy, and patients' expectations for improvement. Each treatment consisted of a 1-hour session once a week for 16 weeks, followed by three booster sessions over the next 3 months. Ten visual analogue scales measured hypochondriacal rituals, fears, and avoidance tactics. On an 18-item cognition questionnaire, patients rated their mean frequency of thoughts (1–5) and their level of belief about having a specific illness (1–100). In addition, several mood questionnaires were included, such as the Beck Anxiety Inventory (Beck et al. 1988), Beck Depression Inventory (Beck et al. 1979), and Hamilton Anxiety Rating Scale (Hamilton 1959). Assessments were conducted at baseline, midtreatment (8 weeks), end of treatment (16 weeks), and at 3-, 6-, and 12-month follow-up.

The dropout rate in this study was only 4%, indicating a high level of patient acceptance of these treatments. Results at 16 weeks showed that both active treatments were more effective in treating hypochondriasis than no treatment, that significant improvement occurred on all hypochondriacal and mood measures, and that significant improvement was maintained by patients in active therapy at 12-month follow-up. Cognitive therapy resulted in a more rapid rate of response than behavioral stress management therapy. At the 8-week and 16-week assessments, cognitive therapy also resulted in a significantly greater improvement in hypochondriasis on most measures than behavioral stress management therapy. In particular, behavioral stress management therapy did not appear to have any effect on the time that patients seriously worried about their health, their level of avoidance of health stressors, and their belief about having an illness. At the follow-ups, however, the gains from cognitive therapy had diminished, whereas the gains from behavioral stress management therapy had been sustained. In other words, although patients in each active therapy group were still significantly better than they had been before treatment, most of the differences between the active treatments themselves were no longer significant. Clark et al. (1998) may have been unable to identify differences between treatments over time because of power problems that arise when the sample size in each treatment group is too small for researchers to detect actual differences between groups.

Because neither active treatment was much better than the other at long-term follow-up in the Clark study, it cannot be concluded that the optimal treatment for hypochondriasis is cognitive therapy. Rather, the improvement experienced by patients in the study may have resulted from the attention they received or from particular beneficial aspects of the behavioral stress management therapy. The behavioral stress management therapy did include valuable behavioral strategies, such as applied relaxation training, which is known to reduce somatic symptoms; stimulus control techniques to reduce worrying time; and exposure to health anxiety cues and situations. Further, the behavioral stress management therapy had a cognitive component in that patients received a detailed alternative explanation for their symptoms. Research that involves separating the attentional from the programmatic aspects of the treatment will help determine which components contribute most to efficacy.

Physiologic Model

Some researchers suggest that people who develop disorders such as hypochondriasis may have lower thresholds for responding physiologically to stressful life events and thus a heightened sensitivity to specific fear cues (Oberhummer et al. 1983). The scientific literature also suggests that people who have a heightened physiological response to anxiety triggers may be more susceptible to anxiety disorders (Eysenck 1979). Gramling et al. (1996) conducted a psychophysiological study using cold pressor and imagery tasks to assess pain perception and stress reactivity in 15 individuals with hypochondriasis and 15 control subjects. Basing the diagnosis of hypochondriasis on the scores obtained from a well-established self-report questionnaire (Illness Attitude Scale), but not necessarily on DSM-IV criteria (American Psychiatric Association 1994), the investigators found that the individuals with hypochondriasis exhibited a significant increase in heart rate and a significant drop in hand temperature compared with the control group. The fact that the individuals with hypochondriasis were physiologically more reactive may have been the result of "hard-wired" constitutional differences or an acquired response learned by means of modeling, reinforcement, or classical conditioning. Kukleta (1991) theorized that people with hypochondriasis have a greater tendency to become more physiologically aroused in the presence of a perceived threat than those without the disorder. Thus, the combination of heightened sensitivity and a specific stressor may result in repetition of distressing thoughts, which subsequently may lead to ritualistic behaviors to reduce the discomfort. Many empirical studies of the psychophysiology of hypochondria are difficult to evaluate because few of the studies used DSM diagnostic criteria, few used clinically ill patients, and psychiatric comorbidity was often not studied.

In a study on somatosensory amplification, Barsky et al. 1995 employed a careful study design to examine whether patients with hypochondriasis were more accurate or more sensitive detectors of their internal bodily states. Sixty patients with DSM-III-R (American Psychiatric Association 1987) hypochondriasis were compared with 60 patients without the disorder using a heartbeat detection test (Barsky et al. 1995). On an objective measure of visceral interoception, there was no difference between the two groups. Of patients with hypochondriasis, 5.5% were able to detect the instant of cardiac contraction compared with 14.0% of the control group ($P = 0.12$). These same hypochondriasis patients, however, had scores on the Somatosensory Amplification Scale that were significantly higher than those of the control subjects, indicating their subjective belief that they were extremely sensitive to normal physiologic sensations and minor bodily symptoms. These results did not change even after controlling for the potentially confounding influences of gender, weight, and state of anxiety. The conclusion from this study is that patients with DSM-III-R hypochondriasis are not more accurately aware of their resting heartbeat than control subjects in the same medical setting. Further research among clinically diagnosed samples using different measures of interoceptive sensitivity will help determine whether patients with hypochondriasis are not more physiologically sensitive to benign bodily sensations.

Treatment of Hypochondriasis

Initial Aspects of Treatment

Establishment of Trust

The first objective is to develop a relationship of trust with the patient and to show an appreciation for the patient's problems. By demonstrating a thoughtful, impartial, and empathic nature through the joining process and reflective listening, the lines of communication are facilitated, and sufficient information can be gathered to make a practical assessment of the patient's problem. Trust is enhanced by validation of the patient's experience of symptoms and by avoiding the use of alarming diagnostic terms. At our somatic disorders treatment program at the New York State Psychiatric Institute, we use the term "heightened illness concern" rather than "hypochondriasis," because the former is a more accurate description of the patient's experience and the latter is often perceived as pejorative. Although these patients are often experienced by others as "difficult" because of their resistance to psychological treatment, frequent medical complaints, and habitual reassurance seeking, it is important for the therapist to be tolerant and sympathetic to make patients feel that their health concerns are being taken seriously.

History Taking

A careful review of the patient's medical work-up not only serves to further strengthen the patient-doctor bond but also may lead to the detection of inadequate work-ups or even an underlying explanation for the patient's particular complaints. Rather than hastily dismissing chronic health complaints as purely a symptom of a psychological disorder, this approach allows the clinician to be sure that an adequate work-up was conducted and provides invaluable information about the initial occurrence, seriousness, and prevalence of the patient's somatic concerns. Only then can the next step be taken in which information is collected about the patient's coping mechanisms, perceptions of problems, and previous therapeutic contacts.

Identification of Stressors

The therapist should attempt to identify any environmental, social, or biological factors that could be maintaining the illness-related fears. A cognitive therapist would emphasize variables that are maintaining the anxiety, whereas a psychodynamic psychotherapist would spend more time exploring experiences that might relate to the patient's current distress. To evaluate a patient's reactions to stressful situations, cognitive therapists may use guided imagery to re-create a real-life difficulty. A therapist can ask the patient to conjure up an image of going to a doctor's office and ask him or her to articulate any fears that come to mind.

Therapists working with patients with hypochondriasis rarely initiate questions with "why," preferring to focus on empirically based questions starting with "how," "when," "where," and "what." This type of inquiry enables the therapist to get a more complete picture of the role of hypochondriasis symptoms in the context of a patient's daily life and to make a more rapid identification of contradictions and distortions in the patient's self-reports. Questions can be phrased accordingly: "What precedes your sporadic bouts of illness phobia?" "When and where are you most likely to feel distressed about your health?" "How do you feel after you remove yourself from an anxiety-provoking situation such as a hospital or doctor's office?" Behavioral methods use the "here-and-now" orientation, targeting specific behaviors, stressing problem solving, and assessing the patient's strengths and weaknesses.

Self-Report Instruments

Self-report instruments, such as diaries in which to express illness fears and write down somatic symptoms, can help the patient observe the waxing and waning of symptoms as stressful events occur. These instruments can also help the therapist objectively assess the severity and complexity of the problem in order to set properly targeted goals. Helpful instruments include the Heightened Illness Concern Diary (Fallon 2001) and the Illness Attitude Scale.

Education

Because patients may be reluctant to engage in treatment for a psychiatric disorder if they consider the problem to be a medical one better solved by physicians, educating patients about how stress, emotions, poor diet, or lack of exercise may trigger real physical symptoms is an essential component of the initial engagement process. We and others have found it helpful to recommend books, written from the patient's perspective, that describe hypochondriasis in its individual and social context as well as providing a clear description of various treatment options. Carla Cantor's book, *Phantom Illness*, serves this purpose well (Cantor 1996).

Cognitive-Behavioral Treatment Strategies

Cognitive Aspects of Cognitive-Behavioral Therapy

The principal aim of cognitive therapy is to unravel the core beliefs underlying the patient's hypochondriacal thoughts. Cognitive therapists help their patients understand that an organic medical disorder is not the only reasonable explanation for highly distressing physical symptoms and that distorted patterns of cognition have problematic emotional and behavioral consequences. In cognitive therapy, patients learn to detect and dispute their irrational beliefs about having a serious illness by discriminating these beliefs from rational alternatives (e.g., statistical probability of having the serious illness, alternative and less-threatening explanations of why they might be experiencing pain) (Salkovskis 1996). Patients need to internalize new rational beliefs by employing cognitive, emotive, and behavioral methods of challenging irrational beliefs—a process they can use throughout their lives.

Awareness of habitual patterns of cognition that reflect underlying dysfunctional cognitive structures or irrational beliefs can be achieved by teaching patients to self-monitor their health concerns and triggering symptoms on a day-to-day basis by keeping a diary of dysfunctional thoughts. Antecedent perceptions and their relationship to ongoing feelings and behaviors can then be more readily identified. Patients are encouraged to challenge their maladaptive thought patterns by listing all the "evidence" supporting their belief that they have a dreaded illness as well as all the evidence that they are not ill. Patients are also asked to examine each of their health complaints and use medical statistics to consider the likelihood that a serious illness actually exists. The patient's need for reassurance also needs to be addressed through a realization that he or she can never be reassured fully, that health risks always exist, and that the risk of serious illness is too insignificant to cause concern. Through rational restructuring methods and attributional retraining, patients can learn how to solve problems effectively and change their dichotomous reasoning, overgeneralizing, and catastrophizing (Warwick and Salkovskis 1989). Over time, their enhanced awareness will lead them to actively challenge their expectations of harmful health consequences (Warwick and Salkovskis 1989).

Educating patients about the merits of limiting maladaptive behavioral reinforcement can be helpful. Although repetitive reassurance seeking, body checks, and doctor visits reduce short-term anxiety, in the long term these behaviors reinforce obsessions, further convincing patients that there will be terrible health consequences if they do not perform their compulsions (Salkovskis and Warwick 1986). A patient of ours with profound hypochondriacal anxiety responded well to clomipramine therapy, to the point that she was able to use the cognitive-behavioral strategies she had learned. For example, in a demonstration of considerable insight, she called to ask us not to accept more than one call from her per week; this self-imposed limit setting worked and she felt less anxious.

Behavioral Aspects of Cognitive-Behavioral Therapy

Exposure.   Exposure to anxiety-provoking stimuli is performed gradually and hierarchically by presenting moderately upsetting stressors, followed by several intermediate stressors and then the most distressing ones (Warwick and Salkovskis 1989). Hierarchies are targeted to expose patients to situations, places, or feelings they often avoid. Treatment sessions frequently include both actual (in vivo) exposure and imaginal exposure (Sisti 1997). In vivo exposure may involve having the patient visit hospitals, come in contact with ill patients, and elicit physical sensations (e.g., pain, dizziness, palpitations) through strenuous activity; providing medical information; and discussing illness (Warwick and Marks 1988). Someone with an AIDS phobia might be desensitized to his or her fears first by walking outside a hospital, then walking inside the hospital, followed by a visit to an AIDS ward. Patients can use imaginal or indirect exposure methods in which they imagine a doctor diagnosing them with a dreaded disease. They can rehearse this doctor-patient interaction by writing it down repeatedly, mentally reviewing the scenario, or listening to an endless loop audiotape of this frightening narration until they habituate to the fear (Sisti 1997).

The patient and therapist work together to develop a list of exposure exercises to be performed during sessions as well as exposure exercises to be done between sessions. Exposure therapy helps provide patients who are experiencing anxiety with insight into their thoughts, images, impulses, physiological symptoms, and self-reported levels of tension. After each exposure session, the therapist carefully examines the patient's specific thoughts and images for distortions, and teaches the patient necessary coping skills. The cognitive component is therefore intricately interwoven with the behavioral (Salkovskis and Warwick 1986).

Successful exposure therapy requires adequate duration, frequency, and comprehensiveness. A prolonged duration of exposure to stressors is needed to achieve a substantial reduction in the level of fear. Shorter exposures raise the risk that the patient will remain uncomfortable and fearful (Foa and Kozak 1986). The frequency of exposure is also consequential because repeated exposure to a stressor results in gradual habituation to the external stimuli, ultimately resulting in a decrease in fear. This "practice makes perfect" phenomenon emphasizes the importance of daily exposure exercises to reduce fear. Comprehensiveness of exposure is necessary to prevent relapse and achieve long-term therapeutic success. All aspects of patients' fears must be addressed, including mood, cognitive distortions, and maladaptive behaviors that enhance their health fears. The therapist may use imaginal exposure by encouraging patients to focus on physiological and behavioral reactions to their fears. In conjunction with in vivo exposure, imaginal exposure helps expose patients to the cognitive components of their fears, thereby maximizing relapse prevention by contributing to the comprehensiveness of treatment (Sisti 1997).

Response-prevention therapy.   One of the earliest reports of response-prevention therapy comes from the work of Shoma Morita, who in the 1920s developed a treatment for hypochondriasis that consisted partly of ignoring patients' hypochondriacal complaints—a type of systematic nonreinforcement (Kitanishi 1990). Because this extinction strategy was used while patients were being cared for by family members in Dr. Morita's home, a message of acceptance and support was conveyed without reinforcing the hypochondriacal reassurance needs.

In contemporary response-prevention therapy, the therapist creates a treatment plan in which the patient is prevented from performing daily rituals. Together the therapist and patient negotiate a reduced number of times the patient is allowed to consult medical books, check his or her body for lumps and bumps, or ask doctors and family for reassurance. In outpatient treatment, it is customarily the patient's responsibility to abide by the treatment plan and abstain from ritualistic behavior. A supervisor, such as a family member or close friend, is often asked to participate in the response-prevention exercises. He or she helps monitor the time and frequency the patient engages in certain behaviors and is often instructed on how often and the manner in which reassurance should be given. Abstinence from rituals and level of supervision vary considerably among different therapies. Although the level of supervision does not seem to significantly affect patient improvement, the strictness of rules appears to affect treatment compliance. The more stringent and detailed the response-prevention instructions are for the patient, the fewer decisions the patient has to make regarding what is normal and what is ritualistic behavior, ultimately resulting in better compliance (Foa and Kozak 1985).

In a retrospective study conducted by Logsdail et al. (1991), 6 (86%) of 7 nondepressed patients whose illness phobia centered on AIDS demonstrated significant improvement after 7–10 sessions of prolonged exposure to obsessional cues and strict prevention of ritualistic behaviors. The therapist accompanied some patients during in vivo and imaginal exposures when necessary. As is the case for the treatment of OCD, the combination of exposure and response prevention is more effective at long-term follow-up than treatments that include only one of these two components. Exposure works by reducing obsessional distress, whereas response prevention aims to reduce rituals (Foa et al. 1984).

Alternative Treatments

Relaxation Therapy

Relaxation therapy is a core technique used in many comprehensive behavioral and stress management interventions. The goal of relaxation therapy is to reduce arousal in both the central nervous system and autonomic nervous system in order to sustain psychological and physical health; this is done through abdominal breathing exercises, progressive muscle relaxation, or visual imagery (Jacobson 1938). Relaxation therapy, which aims to reduce muscle tension, seemingly contradicts the goal of behavioral therapy, which aims to increase physiological arousal to promote habituation to anxiety. However, behavioral therapists often use relaxation techniques between exposure exercises to decrease residual anxiety. Patients are encouraged to practice relaxation during the absence of immediate stressors rather than when they are in the throes of anxiety. Relaxation therapy is cost-effective and relatively risk free. In a controlled study, behavioral stress management therapy using progressive relaxation techniques was shown to be an appropriate and effective therapeutic tool for improving hypochondriasis and mood (Clark et al. 1998).

Relaxation is considered a skill the patient can learn and apply to a variety of situations. This self-initiated coping skill gives the patient the ability to recognize rising levels of tension and to reduce tension through particular exercises. The key components to mastering this skill are rehearsal and self-monitoring.

Relaxation therapy is useful in eliminating conditioned anxiety, which causes insomnia, interpersonal distress, and behavioral problems, as well as in promoting communication in therapy sessions by reducing the patient's tension. If the patient is more relaxed, he or she will be more likely to trust and have confidence in the therapist and consequently be more emotionally expressive. Overall, relaxation therapy can serve as a key component of a treatment plan to manage the physical, emotional, and psychological tension that often accompanies hypochondriasis.

Supportive Psychotherapy

Supportive psychotherapy is nonspecific, but it generally includes reassurance, education, and life-stressor management. Some literature suggests that supportive psychotherapy can be helpful. Kellner (1983) conducted a prospective clinical study using supportive psychotherapy consisting of accurate information about symptoms, education about the role of selective perception of symptoms, repeated medical reassurance, repeated physical examinations, and antianxiety medication as needed. His study showed that 64% of patients experienced significant improvement or full recovery after supportive psychotherapy. Seventy-six percent of the patients who responded to supportive psychotherapy had hypochondriasis for less than 3 years and demonstrated sustained improvement at 2-year follow-up. Kellner's study, however, did not determine conclusively the reason for patients' improvement, because the study did not control for frequency of doctor visits or administration of antianxiety medication.

Fava et al. (2000) randomly assigned 20 patients with DSM-IV hypochondriasis to either explanatory therapy or to a waiting-list control group followed by explanatory therapy. Explanatory therapy led to improvement in both groups as evidenced by a reduction in hypochondriasis, depression, and use of health care services at 6-month follow-up. The therapy consisted of 8 sessions over a 16-week period, each lasting a half hour. During treatment, patients were encouraged to record their worst illness fears in a diary and to write alternative interpretations of their somatic symptoms. Patients were educated about the role of perceived threat and excessive attention in the enhancement or induction of somatic symptoms. Ratings tools included the Illness Attitude Scale, Clinical Interview for Depression, and Rating Scale of Somatic Symptoms. Although the patients who underwent explanatory therapy showed significantly greater improvement than the waiting-list control group on most measures, they still had substantial symptoms at the end of treatment, leading the authors to conclude that "the aim of therapy may be for the patient to regain control over hypochondriacal symptoms rather than to expect their complete disappearance." This observation suggests that explanatory therapy, although helpful, may not lead to as robust a change as evidenced with other treatments, such as pharmacotherapy and cognitive therapy.

Education is a key component of supportive psychotherapy because it can be used to persuade the patient that the primary problem is not an actual medical illness. Patients with excessive health concerns often prefer to be provided with a rationale for why they are experiencing their physical symptoms rather than a confirmation that they do not have any serious health threats. Key to this rationale is a thorough explanation of how emotional triggers, such as family conflict, job stress, low self-esteem, dependency issues, and undetected fears, can lead people to feel physically vulnerable, and hence, worry excessively about potential health problems. By addressing this topic in a compassionate and tolerant manner, the mental health professional avoids undermining the seriousness of the patient's health concerns. When physical complaints are coupled with reasonable explanations, patients may not feel as compelled to seek reassurance (Warwick and Salkovskis 1989). A randomized controlled trial of psychiatric consultation and psychoeducation for patients with unexplained somatic complaints demonstrated the benefit of regular supportive care and office visits focused on reducing somatization (Smith et al. 1986). The same may be true for hypochondriasis.

Practitioners of supportive psychotherapy need to know how much reassurance to offer. They must also try to predict, based on certain character traits, which patients will respond most effectively to reassurance. Patients with serious underlying character pathology may respond to reassurance with rage and aggression because they may feel as if the doctors are undermining their health concerns. Other patients may view reassurance as the glue that strengthens their relationship with the doctor (Starcevic 1990). Some patients require more frequent and comprehensive explanations of their medical status, whereas other patients prefer fewer details (Kessel 1979). Researchers differ considerably in their views about appropriate provision of medical reassurance. Warwick (1992) and Warwick and Salkovskis (1990) believed that repeated reassurance is detrimental because it maintains the mistaken belief that there is a health danger. On the other side of the debate, Kellner (1992), Pilowsky (1983), and Starcevic (1991, 2000) believed that frequent and detailed medical reassurance can be beneficial in helping a patient better manage anxiety related to health concerns. This debate will be resolved only through systematic controlled research.

Pharmacotherapy

Unlike pharmacological approaches for treating hypochondriasis that is secondary to another condition (e.g., depression, panic disorder), pharmacological approaches for treating primary hypochondriasis were considered generally unsuccessful until the 1990s, when reports emerged suggesting that serotonin reuptake inhibitors (SRIs) were particularly effective (see Table 2–2).

> Ms. Q, a 19-year-old college student, had experienced hypochondriacal symptoms since age 8, when her frequent bouts of head pain precipitated a fear that she had cancer. She made fre-

Table 2–2. Pharmacologic trials for treatment of hypochondriasis

Study	N	Design	Evaluation tools	Type of patient	Type(s) of therapy	Results	Comments
Pilowsky 1968	66	Retrospective	Clinical interview	Inpatients with primary hypochondriasis	50% received ECT, 50% received antidepressants	50% of all patients experienced improvement at 2-year follow-up	Good outcome associated with short duration of illness and absence of personality disorder
Wesner and Noyes 1991	10	8-week prospective		Outpatients with DSM-III-R hypochondriasis with good insight	Imipramine (150 mg/day)	100% experienced moderate improvement	Patients with illness phobia had good insight, possibly indicating a distinct subgroup
Fallon et al. 1993	16	12-week prospective	CGI Scale, SCID, Whiteley Index	Nondepressed outpatients with DSM-III-R hypochondriasis	Fluoxetine (20–80 mg/day)	71% responded after 12 weeks	Greater response at 12 weeks than at 6 weeks suggests higher dose or longer treatment is needed
Fallon et al. 1996	25	12-week prospective, controlled	CGI Scale, IAS, SCID, Whiteley Index	Outpatients with DSM-IV hypochondriasis	Fluoxetine (20–80 mg/day) or placebo	80% response rate for fluoxetine group after 6 and 12 weeks, 50%–60% response rate for placebo group	50% of patients treated with fluoxetine were symptom free compared with 20% of patients receiving placebo, suggesting greater efficacy for fluoxetine, but placebo effect cannot be minimized
Fallon 2001	18	10-week prospective, open label	CGI Scale, IAS, SCID, Whiteley Index	Outpatients with DSM-IV hypochondriasis	Fluvoxamine (300 mg/day) after a 2-week placebo run-in	73% of 11 patients who completed 6 weeks of treatment responded	Fluvoxamine may be an effective SSRI for treatment of hypochondriasis

Note. CGI = Clinical Global Improvement; IAS = Illness Attitude Scale; SCID = Structured Clinical Interview for DSM-IV.

quent visits to the pediatrician for evaluation, magnetic resonance imaging (MRI), computed tomography (CT), and reassurance. Ms. Q's symptoms became particularly distressing at age 18, when she developed stomach aches, which led to the fear that she had appendicitis; a skin rash, which led to the fear that she had cancer; and head pain, which led to the conviction that her death was imminent. She experienced a rapidly escalating sense of terror. No identifiable stressor was evident before Ms. Q's condition worsened. Brief psychotherapy was of little help, and her illness fears were accompanied later by depressed mood. Ms. Q was treated with an SRI, citalopram (20 mg/day). After the first few weeks of treatment, her somatic sensations and fears worsened until, one morning, she awakened to find almost complete resolution of these symptoms. This resolution was sustained during the following 6 months as Ms. Q continued to take medication. Ms. Q had no history of OCD, primary major depression, or panic disorder. She reported no childhood history of trauma, interpersonal loss, or significant illnesses in those close to her.

Therapeutic options for this young woman could have included more intensive psychodynamic psychotherapy to explore unrecognized conflicts, cognitive-behavioral therapy to address her irrational appraisal of threat from bodily symptoms, and/or pharmacotherapy to address her immediate symptoms of profound anxiety and depression. The pharmacotherapy led to a rapid improvement that was sustained over time. Further evaluation of this woman revealed a childhood characterized by considerable emotional neglect. Exploratory psychodynamic psychotherapy was recommended. Based on pharmacologic studies of depression, this woman was advised to continue taking the SRI for at least a full year.

Pharmacotherapy for Secondary Hypochondriasis

Major depression. Kellner et al. (1986a) reported that 4 weeks of treatment with amitriptyline (100–300 mg/day) was effective in reducing hypochondriacal concerns among 20 consecutive nonpsychotic inpatients with DSM-III (American Psychiatric Association 1980) melancholic major depression, one-third of whom had scores on the Illness Attitude Scale that were characteristic of patients with hypochondriasis before treatment.

Panic disorder. Noyes et al. (1986) reported that pharmacologic treatment of 60 patients with panic disorder and agoraphobia resulted in a diminution of panic attacks as well as a significant decrease in hypochondriasis, as measured by the Illness Behavior Questionnaire dimensions of disease fear, disease conviction, and bodily preoccupation.

Obsessive-compulsive disorder. Bodkin and White (1989) reported that clonazepam was very helpful in ameliorating a man's OCD symptoms and hypochondriasis about AIDS. Fallon et al. (1991) reported that fluoxetine at doses of 60 mg/day, but not 20–40 mg/day, were effective in reducing DSM-III-R hypochondriasis and OCD. Similar to the pharmacotherapy of OCD, this case suggested that hypochondriasis patients with a stronger obsessional component may preferentially respond to the higher doses of fluoxetine often needed to treat OCD successfully.

Delusional disorder, somatic subtype. This disorder, also known as "atypical psychosis" or "monosymptomatic hypochondriacal psychosis," refers to hypochondriasis of delusional intensity. Often the disease the patient fears he or she has is rare, such as spongiform encephalitis (mad cow disease). Case reports suggest that antipsychotic medications, such as haloperidol (Fishbain et al. 1992), pimozide (Lippert 1986; Scarone and Gambini 1991), and thioridazine (Scarone and Gambini 1991), may reduce convictions of delusional intensity to nonpsychotic proportions.

Pharmacotherapy for Primary Hypochondriasis

In a retrospective study, Pilowsky (1968) identified 66 psychiatric inpatients with primary hypochondriasis, half of whom had been given either electroconvulsive therapy or antidepressants. Half of the patients had good outcome after 2 years, with good prognosis associated with a shorter duration of hypochondriacal fears and the absence of a comorbid personality disorder.

Imipramine. Imipramine, a medication that exhibits both serotonergic and noradrenergic reuptake inhibition, has been reported to be effective in case reports and a small open series. In a case report, Lippert (1986) found that 150 mg/day of imipramine was helpful for a man who, for 3 months, had hypochondriasis about AIDS compounded by major depression. In a small open series, Wesner and Noyes (1991) conducted an 8-week prospective open trial of imipramine at a mean final dose of 144 mg/day and reported that all patients showed at least moderate improvement by 4 weeks, with one patient symptom free. Using the data from the Fallon et al. (1996) placebo-controlled fluoxetine study and the Wesner and Noyes data on imipramine, a comparison of virtually symptom-free patients showed the following: 50% of patients had been given fluoxetine, 20% placebo, and 12.5% imipramine. Although these results suggest a lack of effectiveness of imipramine, a direct comparison with more selective serotonin reuptake inhibitors (SSRIs) and placebo in a larger number of patients will help determine whether imipramine is effective in treating hypochondriasis.

Clomipramine. Clomipramine has been reported as being helpful in treating hypochondriasis in several case reports, at doses ranging from 25 mg/day (Kamlana and Gray 1988) to 200 mg/day (Stone 1993). In Stone's report, a 31-year-old man with a 10-year history of primary hypochondriasis did not show improvement despite many previous pharmacologic treatments, including treatment with benzodiazepines, mood stabilizers, beta-blockers, antipsychotics, and tricyclic antidepressants.

Fluvoxamine. Fluvoxamine was reported to be effective for treating hypochondriasis in a case report and an uncontrolled open-label trial. In the case report (Fallon et al. 1996), a 38-year-old woman experienced hypochondriacal fears of breast cancer, engaged in repeated self-checking, and underwent medical evaluations for 3 years. The woman experienced no improvement with a 12-week trial of fluoxetine (80 mg/day); however, she did experience improvement after 8 weeks of treatment with fluvoxamine (300 mg/day). This progress was sustained over the ensuing 3 years. This case suggested that failure to respond to one SSRI does not preclude response to a different SSRI.

In a 10-week open-label trial of fluvoxamine with a 2-week placebo run-in (Fallon 2001), patients completed the Heightened Illness Concern Diary, measures of hypochondriasis (Analog Scale,

Whiteley Index, Illness Attitude Scale), and a measure of functional status (Medical Outcomes Study 36-Item Short-Form Health Survey [SF-36]) before treatment with fluvoxamine, which was increased gradually to 300 mg/day. In this study, 4 (22%) of 18 patients were excluded during the placebo run-in phase either because of marked improvement or noncompliance with the medication or study visits. Three patients discontinued treatment before 6 weeks. Eight (73%) of 11 patients who completed the minimum treatment of at least 6 weeks responded to treatment and 8 (57%) of 14 patients given active fluvoxamine responded. Even though these results suggest that fluvoxamine may be effective for treating hypochondriasis, the greater than 25% dropout rate in active treatment suggests that pharmacotherapy may be less acceptable to patients than psychotherapy. This suggestion is supported by a 4.6% dropout rate reported by Clark et al. (1998) in their study of cognitive therapy and behavioral stress management therapy, as well as by Walker et al. (1999) in an opinion survey, which indicated that 17 (74%) of 23 patients with DSM-IV hypochondriasis preferred cognitive-behavioral therapy to pharmacotherapy.

Fluoxetine.   Fluoxetine for the treatment of hypochondriasis has been well studied. Two separate case reports (Fallon et al. 1991; Viswanathan and Paradis 1991) suggested that fluoxetine (40–80 mg/day) is beneficial for patients with treatment-refractory hypochondriasis. Each of the patients in these case reports did not respond to previous treatments, including psychotherapy (which included behavioral therapy in one case), nonserotonergic antidepressants, antianxiety agents, and antipsychotic medications.

Fallon et al. (1993) reported the results of a 12-week open-label trial of fluoxetine for 16 patients with hypochondriasis without major depression, with doses starting at 20 mg/day, increasing every 2 weeks by 20 mg/day as tolerated and needed, to 80 mg/day. Only 2 patients dropped out of the trial during the initial weeks of active medication treatment, and 14 completed all 12 weeks. Among patients who completed treatment, the response rate at 12 weeks (71.4%) was twice the rate at 6 weeks (35.7%), suggesting that longer courses of therapy might be needed for hypochondriasis. Alternatively, because the mean dose of fluoxetine was higher at 12 weeks than at 6 weeks (52 mg/day versus 39 mg/day), the critical factor may be medication dose rather than duration. Four of the patients who responded to fluoxetine were virtually symptom free at the end of treatment. Patients with primary hypochondriasis appeared to respond at a higher rate than patients with hypochondriasis complicated by another major comorbid Axis I disorder: 6 (86%) of 7 patients and 4 (57%) of 7 patients, respectively. Although improvement occurred in nearly all measures of hypochondriasis and mood, there was no statistical improvement in bodily preoccupation.

Fallon et al. (1996) reported the results of a mid-study analysis of the first 25 patients to enter a double-blind 12-week placebo-controlled study of fluoxetine for DSM-IV hypochondriasis, with doses starting at 20 mg/day and increasing as needed to 80 mg/day. During the 2-week placebo run-in, 5 patients were excluded either because of a placebo response or noncompliance with the protocol. Of the 20 patients assigned randomly to placebo or fluoxetine, 16 (80%) completed a minimum treatment of 6 weeks and 15 (75%) completed the full 12 weeks. Eight (80%) of 10 patients randomized to fluoxetine responded at 6 and 12 weeks versus a placebo response of 3 (50%) of 6 patients at 6 weeks and 3 (60%) of 5 patients at 12 weeks on the Clinical Global Improvement (CGI) Scale. These response rates, although high for fluoxetine at 6 and 12 weeks, also indicated a robust placebo response at 6 and 12 weeks, respectively. When the data were reexamined to rate response as a score of "very much improved" on the CGI Scale (virtually symptom free), the response rate was higher for fluoxetine than placebo at 12 weeks: 5 (50%) of 10 fluoxetine-randomized patients versus 1 (20%) of 5 placebo-randomized patients. This mid-study analysis of a double-blind placebo-controlled study suggested preferential efficacy for fluoxetine but also raised critical questions about the nonspecific therapeutic effects of placebo and patient-clinician encounters. A similar concern emerged from the Clark et al. (1998) study of cognitive therapy versus behavioral stress management therapy for treating hypochondriasis.

Therapeutic Suggestions for Pharmacologic Treatment

Patients with hypochondriasis who are considering a medication trial benefit from a careful explanation of how the medicine might reduce illness obsessions and distress over bodily symptoms by acting on the neurochemistry of the brain, correcting an imbalance that would otherwise allow the hypochondriasis to continue. Because patients with hypochondriasis are often fearful of the unknown long-term consequences of medication, an honest and open discussion about the risks and benefits of medication treatment should be conducted, with the physician being careful not to provide excessive detail that would only further frighten the patient. As part of the discussion of pharmacotherapy, the physician should emphasize that therapeutic action may take 6 weeks or longer and that initial side effects often decrease after the first several weeks.

Although pharmacotherapy may not be the preferred choice of treatment for most people with hypochondriasis, 70–80% of patients participating in hypochondriasis trials appear to benefit from them.

Conclusion

Numerous options exist for treating hypochondriasis. Although researchers have not yet identified the exact mechanism of efficacy of various treatments nor which treatments work best for particular patients, it is clear that many patients with hypochondriasis can benefit from serotonergic pharmacotherapy and cognitive-behavioral psychotherapy. Controlled research has demonstrated that cognitive-behavioral therapy is significantly more effective than stress management therapy at short-term assessment. Stress management therapy or explanatory/supportive therapy without response-prevention behavioral therapy may also be helpful, but may be less effective than cognitive-behavioral therapy. The role of exploratory psychodynamic psychotherapy will be determined only after controlled inquiry into its effectiveness for treatment of hypochondriasis. No controlled studies that demonstrate either the efficacy or inefficacy of a medication over placebo have been published yet. Although pharmacotherapy reports appear promising, with rates of improvement up to 80%, the strong placebo response suggests that some of the improvement may be the result of other aspects of the therapy, such as self-monitoring and the attention and education the patient receives from the clinician. Future research needs to clarify the historical and phenomenological factors that will guide the clinician as he or she recommends one treatment over another. Furthermore, comparison studies will help determine whether the optimal choice of treatment is psychotherapy alone, pharmacotherapy alone, or the two combined.

References

American Psychiatric Association: Diagnostic and Statistical Manual of Mental Disorders, 3rd Edition. Washington, DC, American Psychiatric Association, 1980

American Psychiatric Association: Diagnostic and Statistical Manual of Mental Disorders, 3rd Edition, Revised. Washington, DC, American Psychiatric Association, 1987

American Psychiatric Association: Diagnostic and Statistical Manual of Mental Disorders, 4th Edition. Washington, DC, American Psychiatric Association, 1994

Barsky AJ: Hypochondriacal patients, their physicians, and their medical care. J Gen Intern Med 6:413–419, 1991

Barsky AJ: Hypochondriasis and obsessive compulsive disorder. Psychiatr Clin North Am 15:791–801, 1992

Barsky AJ, Wyshak G, Klemran GI: Transient hypochondriasis. Arch Gen Psychiatry 47:746–752, 1990

Barsky AJ, Brener J, Coeytaux RR, et al: Accurate awareness of heartbeat in hypochondriacal and non-hypochondriacal patients. J Psychosom Res 39:489–497, 1995

Barsky AJ, Bailey ED, Fama JM, et al: Predictors of remission in DSM hypochondriasis. Compr Psychiatry 41:179–183, 2000

Beck AT, Emery G: Anxiety Disorders and Phobias: A Cognitive Perspective. New York, Basic Books, 1985

Beck AT, Rusk AJ, Shaw BF, et al: Cognitive Therapy of Depression. New York, Guilford, 1979

Beck AT, Epstein N, Brown G, et al: An inventory for measuring clinical anxiety: psychometric properties. J Consult Clin Psychol 56:893–897, 1988

Berrios GE: Hypochondriasis: history of the concept, in Hypochondriasis: Modern Perspectives on an Ancient Malady. Edited by Starcevic V and Lipsitt D. New York, Oxford University Press, 2001, pp 3–20

Bienvenu OJ, Samuels JF, Riddle MA, et al: The relationship of obsessive-compulsive disorder to possible spectrum disorders: results from a family study. Biol Psychiatry 48:287–293, 2000

Bodkin JA, White K: Clonazepam in the treatment of obsessive compulsive disorder associated with panic disorder in one patient. J Clin Psychiatry 50:265–266, 1989

Bouman TK, Visser S: Cognitive and behavioural treatment of hypochondriasis. Psychother Psychosom 67:214–221, 1998

Cantor C: Phantom Illness: Recognizing, Understanding, and Overcoming Hypochondria. New York, Houghton Mifflin, 1996

Carrns A: Cyberchondriacs get what goes around on the Internet now. The Wall Street Journal, October 5, 1999, p A1

Cheyne G: The English Malady, or, A Treatise of Nervous Diseases of All Kinds, As Spleen, Vapours, Lowness of Spirits, Hypochondriacal, and Hysterical Distempers, Etc. London, J Strachan, 1733

Clark DM, Salkovskis PM, Hackmann A, et al: Two psychological treatments for hypochondriasis. A randomised controlled trial. Br J Psychiatry 173:218–225, 1998

Dollard J, Miller NE: Personality and Psychotherapy: An Analysis in Terms of Learning, Thinking and Culture. New York, McGraw-Hill, 1950

Eysenck HJ: The conditioning model of neurosis. Behav Brain Sci 2:155–199, 1979

Fabre D (ed): Maladies de l'encéphale, maladies mentales, maladies nerveuses, in Bibliothèque du Médecin-Practicien, Vol 9. Paris, Bailliere, 1847

Fallon BA: Pharmacologic strategies for hypochondriasis, in Hypochondriasis: Modern Perspectives on an Ancient Malady. Edited by Starcevic V, Lipsitt D. New York, Oxford University Press, 2001, pp 329–351

Fallon BA, Javitch JA, Hollander E, et al: Hypochondriasis and obsessive compulsive disorder: overlaps in diagnosis and treatment. J Clin Psychiatry 52:457–460, 1991

Fallon BA, Liebowitz MR, Salman E, et al: Fluoxctine for hypochondriacal patients without major depression. J Clin Psychopharmacol 13:438–441, 1993

Fallon BA, Schneier FR, Marshall R, et al: The pharmacotherapy of hypochondriasis. Psychopharmacol Bull 32:607–611, 1996

Fallon BA, Qureshi AI, Laje G, et al: Hypochondriasis and its relationship to obsessive-compulsive disorder. Psychiatr Clin North Am 23: 605–616, 2000

Fava GA, Grandi S, Rafanelli C, et al: Explanatory therapy in hypochondriasis. J Clin Psychiatry 61:317–322, 2000

Fishbain DA, Barsky S, Goldberg M: Monosymptomatic hypochondriacal psychosis: belief of contracting rabies. Int J Psychiatry Med 22:3–9, 1992

Foa EB, Kozak MJ: Treatment of anxiety disorders: implications for psychopathology, in Emotion and Therapeutic Change. Edited by Tuma AH, Maser JD. New York, Guilford, 1985, pp 21–49

Foa EB, Kozak MJ: Emotional processing of fear: exposure to corrective information. Psychol Bull 99:20–35, 1986

Foa EB, Steketee G, Grayson JB, et al: Deliberate exposure and blocking of obsessive-compulsive rituals: immediate and long-term effects. Behavior Therapy 15:450–472, 1984

Freud S: On narcissism: an introduction (1914), in The Standard Edition of the Complete Psychological Works of Sigmund Freud, Vol 14. Translated and edited by Strachey J. London, Hogarth Press, 1955, pp 67–102

Freud S: The ego and the id (1923), in The Standard Edition of the Complete Psychological Works of Sigmund Freud, Vol 19. Translated and edited by Strachey J. London, Hogarth Press, 1961, pp 1–66

Goldstein SE, Birnbom F: Hypochondriasis and the elderly. J Am Geriatr Soc 24:150–154, 1976

Gramling SE, Clawson EP, McDonald MK: Perceptual and cognitive abnormality model of hypochondriasis: amplification and physiological reactivity in women. Psychosom Med 58:423–431, 1996

Guislain J: Lecons orales sur les phrenopathies, ou traite theorique et pratique des maladies mentales. Belgium, L Hebbelynck, 1852

Hamilton M: The assessment of anxiety states by rating. Br J Med Psychol 32:50–55, 1959

Jacobson E: Progressive Relaxation. Chicago, University of Chicago Press, 1938

Kamlana SH, Gray P: Fear of AIDS (letter). Br J Psychiatry 15:1291, 1988

Kellner R: The prognosis of treated hypochondriasis: a clinical study. Acta Psychiatr Scand 67:69–79, 1983

Kellner R: Abridged Manual of the Illness Attitude Scales. Albuquerque, New Mexico, University of New Mexico, 1987

Kellner R: The treatment of hypochondriasis: to reassure or not to reassure? The case for reassurance. International Review of Psychiatry 4:71–75, 1992

Kellner R, Fava GA, Lisansky J, et al: Hypochondriacal fears and beliefs in DSM-III melancholia. Changes with amitriptyline. J Affect Disord 10:21–26, 1986a

Kellner R, Slocumb JC, Wiggins RG, et al: The relationship of hypochondriacal fears and beliefs to anxiety and depression. Psychiatric Medicine 4:15–24, 1986b

Kenyon FE: Hypochondriasis: a clinical study. Br J Psychiatry 110:478–488, 1964

Kessel N: Reassurance. Lancet 1:1128–1133, 1979

Kitanishi K: Morita therapy from a transcultural psychiatric view. Journal of Morita Therapy 1:190–194, 1990

Kukleta M: Psychophysiological mechanisms in hypochondriasis. Homeostasis in Health and Disease 33:7–12, 1991

Ladee GA: Hypochondriacal Syndromes. New York, Elsevier, 1966

Lippert GP: Excessive concern about AIDS in two bisexual men. Can J Psychiatry 31:63–65, 1986

Lipsitt DR: Psychodynamic perspectives on hypochondriasis, in Hypochondriasis: Modern Perspectives on an Ancient Malady. Edited by Starcevic V, Lipsitt D. New York, Oxford University Press, 2001, pp 183–201

Logsdail S, Lovell K, Warwick H, et al: Behavioural treatment of AIDS-focused illness phobia. Br J Psychiatry 159:422–425, 1991

Miller D, Acton TMG, Hedge B: The worried well: their identification and management. J R Coll Physicians Lond 22:158–165, 1988

Noyes R, Reich J, Clancy J, et al: Reduction in hypochondriasis with treatment of panic disorder. Br J Psychiatry 149:631–635, 1986

Oberhummer I, Sachs G, Stellamor M: A comparison of psychophysiological reaction patterns in hypochondriacal and obsessive compulsive patients. Zeitschrift für Klinische Psychologie. Forschung und Praxis 12(2, Pt 2):113–125, 1983

Pilowsky I: Dimensions of hypochondriasis. Br J Psychiatry 113:89–93, 1967

Pilowsky I: The response to treatment in hypochondriacal disorders. Aust N Z J Psychiatry 2:88–94, 1968

Pilowsky I: Hypochondriasis, in Handbook of Psychiatry, Vol 4. Edited by Russell GE, Hersov L. Cambridge, Cambridge University Press, 1983

Salkovskis PM: Frontiers of Cognitive Therapy. New York, Guilford, 1996

Salkovskis PM, Clark DM: Panic and hypochondriasis. Advances in Behaviour Research and Therapy 15:23–48, 1993

Salkovskis PM, Warwick HM: Morbid preoccupations, health anxiety and reassurance: a cognitive-behavioural approach to hypochondriasis. Behav Res Ther 24:597–602,1986

Savage G: Hypochondriasis and insanity, in A Dictionary of Psychological Medicine, Vol 1. Edited by Tuke DH. London, J & A Churchill, 1892

Scarone S, Gambini O: Delusional hypochondriasis: nosographic evaluation, clinical course and therapeutic outcome of 5 cases. Psychopathology 24:179–184, 1991

Sisti M: Hypochondriasis, in Practicing Cognitive Therapy: A Guide to Interventions. Edited by Leahy R. Northvale, NJ, Jason Aronson, 1997, pp 169–191

Smeets G, de Jong PJ, Mayer B: If you suffer from a headache, then you have a brain tumour: domain-specific reasoning "bias" and hypochondriasis. Behav Res Ther 38:763–776, 2000

Smith GR, Monson RA, Ray DC: Psychiatric consultation in somatization disorder: a randomized controlled study. N Engl J Med 314: 1407–1413, 1986

Starcevic V: Role of reassurance and psychopathology in hypochondriasis. Psychiatry 53:383–395, 1990

Starcevic V: Reassurance and treatment of hypochondriasis. Gen Hosp Psychiatry 13:122–127, 1991

Starcevic V: Reassurance therapy, in Hypochondriasis: Modern Perspectives on an Ancient Malady. Edited by Starcevic V, Lipsitt D. New York, Oxford University Press, 2001, pp 291– 313

Stern R, Fernandez M: Group cognitive and behavioral treatment for hypochondriasis. BMJ 303:1229–1231, 1991

Stone AB: Treatment of hypochondriasis with clomipramine (letter). J Clin Psychiatry 54:5, 1993

Visser S, Bouman TK: Cognitive-behavioural approaches in the treatment of hypochondriasis: six single case cross-over studies. Behav Res Ther 30:301–306, 1992

Viswanathan R, Paradis C: Treatment of cancer phobia with fluoxetine (letter). Am J Psychiatry 148:1090, 1991

Walker J, Vincent N, Furer P, et al: Treatment preference in hypochondriasis. J Behav Ther Exp Psychiatry 30:251–258, 1999

Warwick H: The treatment of hypochondriasis: to reassure or not to reassure? Provision of appropriate and effective reassurance. International Review of Psychiatry 4:76–80, 1992

Warwick HM, Marks IM: Behavioural treatment of illness phobia and hypochondriasis. A pilot study of 17 cases. Br J Psychiatry 152:239–241, 1988

Warwick HM, Salkovskis PM: Hypochondriasis, in Cognitive Therapy in Clinical Practice: An Illustrative Casebook. Edited by Scott J, Williams J, Mark G, et al. London, Routledge, 1989, pp 78–102

Warwick HM, Salkovskis PM: Hypochondriasis. Behav Res Ther 28: 105–117, 1990

Warwick HM, Clark DM, Cobb AM, et al: A controlled trial of cognitive-behavioural treatment of hypochondriasis. Br J Psychiatry 169:189–195, 1996

Wesner RB, Noyes R Jr: Imipramine: an effective treatment for illness phobia. J Affect Disord 22:43–48, 1991

Willis T: The London Practice of Physick. London, Thomas Basset, 1685

World Health Organization: International Classification of Diseases, 9th Revision. Geneva, World Health Organization, 1977

Chapter 3

Body Dysmorphic Disorder

Katharine A. Phillips, M.D.

Body dysmorphic disorder (BDD) is an intriguing and relatively common somatoform disorder that has been described around the world for more than a century (Phillips 1991). BDD often causes severe distress and notably impaired functioning, and it can lead to suicide. However, this disorder is typically underrecognized in clinical settings.

BDD is defined in DSM-IV as a preoccupation with an imagined defect in appearance; if a slight physical anomaly is present, the person's concern is markedly excessive (American Psychiatric Association 1994). The preoccupation causes clinically significant distress or impairment in social, occupational, or other important areas of functioning, and it cannot be better accounted for by another mental disorder, such as anorexia nervosa. Although BDD is classified as a somatoform disorder, its delusional variant is classified as a psychotic disorder (a type of delusional disorder, somatic type).

History

BDD has long been described in the European and Japanese literature under a variety of rubrics, most often "dysmorphophobia," a term coined by Enrico Morselli more than 100 years ago (Morselli 1891; Phillips 1991). At the turn of the century, Janet (1903) and Kraepelin (1909–1915) described BDD, emphasizing the extreme shame that BDD patients experience. Janet described a young woman who worried that she would never be loved because she was "ugly and ridiculous" and who for 5 years confined herself to a tiny apartment that she rarely left.

Other terms used to describe BDD over the years include "dermatologic hypochondriasis," "beauty hypochondria" (*schönheitshypochondrie*), and "one who is worried about being ugly" (*hässlichkeitskümmerer*) (Phillips 1991). BDD had a consistent presence in the European literature but was generally absent from the American literature and was not included in DSM-I or DSM-II. It first entered U.S. nosology in DSM-III, but only as an example of an atypical somatoform disorder and without diagnostic criteria (American Psychiatric Association 1980). BDD was first accorded separate diagnostic status in DSM-III-R (American Psychiatric Association 1987). Despite its rich historical tradition, BDD has received little investigation until recently.

Prevalence

BDD appears relatively common in clinical settings. In a study in a dermatology setting, 12% of patients screened positive for BDD (Phillips et al. 2000b). In cosmetic surgery settings, rates of 6%, 7%, and 15% have been reported (Ishigooka et al. 1998; Sarwer et al. 1998a, 1998b). Reported rates of BDD are 8%–37% in patients with obsessive-compulsive disorder (OCD) (Brawman-Mintzer et al. 1995; Hollander et al. 1993; Phillips et al. 1998b; Piggott et al. 1994; Simeon et al. 1995; Wilhelm et al. 1997), 11%–13% in patients with social phobia (Brawman-Mintzer et al. 1995; Wilhelm et al. 1997), 26% in patients with trichotillomania (Soriano et al. 1996), and 14%–42% in patients with atypical major depression (Perugi et al. 1998; Phillips et al. 1996a). In one study on atypical depression, BDD was more than twice as common as OCD (Phillips et al. 1996a), and in another study (Perugi et al. 1998), BDD was more common than many other disorders, including OCD, social phobia, simple phobia, generalized anxiety disorder, bulimia nervosa, and substance abuse or dependence. Studies in the general population have reported rates of 0.7% (Faravelli et al. 1997), 1.1% (Bienvenu et al. 2000), 2.2% (Mayville et al. 1999), and 13% (Biby 1998).

BDD is underrecognized, however. Many patients receive non-psychiatric treatment, such as surgery (Fukuda 1977), leaving their

BDD unrecognized. In addition, patients are usually ashamed of their symptoms and reluctant to reveal them (Phillips 1996a). In a study of 17 inpatients with BDD, BDD symptoms were noted in only 5 patient charts and no patient received the diagnosis, despite the fact that BDD was a significant problem in all cases and, in some, the major reason for hospitalization (Phillips et al. 1993). In studies of general outpatients (Zimmerman and Mattia 1998) and outpatients with depression (Phillips et al. 1996a), BDD was missed by the clinician in every case.

Clinical Features

Demographic Characteristics

The mean age of patients in published clinical series on BDD is generally the early to mid-30s (Phillips and Diaz 1997), although the reported age varies widely, from 5 to 80 years. In the largest published series on DSM-IV BDD ($N = 188$), 51% of patients were men (Phillips and Diaz 1997). Other studies have had a preponderance of men (Fukuda 1977; Hollander et al. 1993) or women (Rosen et al. 1995; Veale et al. 1996a), although referral biases are evident in some of these reports, perhaps accounting for these findings. A majority of patients had never been married, and a relatively high percentage were unemployed (Phillips and Diaz 1997).

Appearance Preoccupations

Individuals with BDD are preoccupied with the idea that some aspect of their appearance is unattractive, deformed, ugly, or "not right," when the perceived flaw is actually minimal or nonexistent (Phillips et al. 1993). Some patients describe themselves as hideous, repulsive, or looking like the Elephant Man (Phillips 1996a). Preoccupations usually involve the face or head, most often the skin, hair, or nose (e.g., acne, scarring, pale or red skin, thinning hair, a large or crooked nose). However, any body part can be the focus of concern, and patients typically worry about three or four body areas over the course of their illness (Phillips et al. 1993). In some cases, individuals with BDD report disliking their overall appearance or say they are generally ugly, because they dislike so many body areas or are too embarrassed to discuss specific parts. Concern with bodily asymmetry (e.g., "uneven" buttocks) is common (Phillips 1996a).

Patients with BDD typically think about their perceived flaws for 3–8 hours a day (Phillips 1996a). As Ladee (1966, p. 324) wrote: "The preoccupation is so exclusively centered on one aspect of the bodily appearance, which is experienced as deformed, repulsive, unacceptable, or ridiculous, that the whole of one's existence is dominated by this preoccupation and nothing else has any significance any more." The thoughts are usually difficult to resist or control and are very distressing, as noted by Morselli (1891), who pointed out that "the dysmorphophobic patient is really miserable." Such patients have low self-esteem (Rosen and Ramirez 1998) and are rejection sensitive (Phillips et al. 1996a). Clinical observations suggest that they also have prominent feelings of defectiveness, unworthiness, embarrassment, and shame (Phillips 1996a).

Insight

Before treatment, most patients have poor insight or are delusional, not recognizing that the flaw they perceive is actually minimal or nonexistent. One study (*N* = 100) found that more than half of patients were delusional for a significant period of time (Phillips et al. 1994). However, insight may shift in some patients; therefore, their degree of delusionality may vary over time (Phillips and McElroy 1993). Clinical experience suggests that stress and social exposure, for example, may cause some patients to have less insight.

A majority of patients have ideas or delusions of reference, thinking that other people take special notice of the supposed defect, perhaps staring at it, talking about it, or mocking it (Phillips et al. 1993). Referential thinking can be a prominent aspect of the clinical picture and can significantly contribute to the social isolation that BDD usually causes.

Body Image

Body image is clearly an important aspect of BDD, but has received little investigation. In one study, patients with BDD were less satisfied with their body image than control subjects and were more likely to feel that their body was unacceptable (Hardy 1982). Patients' views of their appearance may be based in abnormal sensory (perceptual) processing or in attitudinal/cognitive-evaluative dissatisfaction. Preliminary empirical reports suggest that BDD patients may not have deficits in sensory processing, but to the contrary, may have unusually good discriminatory ability. In one report, BDD patients more accurately assessed facial proportions than control subjects or cosmetic surgery patients (Thomas and Goldberg 1995). Another study similarly found that BDD patients had a more accurate perception of nose size and shape than a control group (Jerome 1991). In a neuropsychological study, individuals with BDD overfocused on minor and irrelevant stimuli (Deckersbach et al. 2000), suggesting that their appearance-related beliefs may arise from overfocusing on minimal appearance flaws (isolated details rather than overall appearance), causing a visual attention bias.

Compulsive Behaviors

Nearly all individuals with BDD perform repetitive, time-consuming, and compulsive behaviors (Phillips et al. 1994). The usual intent is to examine, improve, seek reassurance about, or hide the perceived defect. Common behaviors are comparing one's appearance with that of others; excessively checking the perceived flaw directly in mirrors or in other reflecting surfaces (e.g., windows); excessively grooming (e.g., applying makeup or tweezing, styling, or cutting hair); seeking reassurance about the perceived flaw or attempting to convince others of its ugliness; and camouflaging (e.g., with hair, a wig, makeup, body position, sunglasses, a hat or other clothing). To hide their faces, some patients wear a mask or hood over their heads.

Other BDD-related behaviors include dieting, excessive exercising, touching or measuring the body part, buying excessive amounts of beauty products, changing clothes repeatedly, and seeking surgery or medical treatment (Phillips 1996a). Men with muscle dysmorphia may use anabolic steroids (Pope et al. 1997, 2000). Patients can be very creative in an effort to diminish their suffering. One woman repeatedly tensed and untensed her facial muscles to make them less limp, and another pushed on her eyeballs to change their shape. To make his face look fuller, a man with BDD slept without a pillow, ate large amounts of food, and drank more than 3 gal of water a day (Phillips 1996a).

Compulsive skin picking is a recognized symptom of BDD (Phillips and Taub 1995). One-third of individuals with this disorder pick their skin in hopes of improving its appearance. Because this behavior is difficult to resist and typically occurs for hours a day, it may cause noticeable skin lesions, especially if implements such as needles or razor blades are used. In more extreme cases, this behavior can be life-threatening, as in the case of a woman who picked at her neck and exposed her carotid artery, requiring emergency surgery (O'Sullivan et al. 1999).

Comorbidity

Most patients with BDD seen in psychiatric settings have other mental disorders. The disorder most often comorbid with BDD is major depression. In one study, a rate of approximately 60% and a lifetime rate of more than 80% was reported (Phillips and Diaz 1997). This study found that BDD usually began before depression, with the depressive symptoms often appearing secondary to BDD. It also found that other commonly comorbid disorders are social phobia, with a lifetime rate of 38%; substance use disorders, with a lifetime rate of 36%; and OCD, with a lifetime rate of 30%. Other studies have reported lower comorbidity rates (Veale et al. 1996a), which may reflect the treatment setting, referral sources, or other factors. Reported rates of a personality disorder in BDD patients seen in psychiatric settings range from 57% to 100%, with avoidant personality disorder most common (Neziroglu et al. 1996; Phillips and McElroy 2000; Veale et al. 1996a).

Complications

Patients with BDD typically experience severe distress over their perceived appearance flaws. Referential thinking, anxiety caused by BDD-related behaviors, and feelings of rejection and social isolation all appear to contribute to this distress. DeMarco et al.

(1998) found that BDD outpatients ($N = 78$) had markedly high levels of perceived stress, with scores on a measure of perceived stress notably higher than those of population norms and most clinical samples. Perceived stress scores were significantly correlated with BDD symptom severity.

Although functioning varies, nearly all individuals with BDD experience impairment in social and academic or occupational functioning (Phillips et al. 1993). They may avoid dating and other social interactions, have few or no friends, or get divorced because of BDD. Impairment in academic or occupational functioning is common and may be caused by poor concentration caused by BDD obsessions, time-consuming BDD-related behaviors, or self-consciousness about being seen. In a series of 33 children and adolescents with BDD, 18% had dropped out of school because of BDD (Albertini and Phillips 1999). In a series of adults with BDD, 8% were on disability primarily because of BDD (K. A. Phillips, unpublished data). More than a quarter of these patients had been completely housebound for at least 1 week, and more than half had been hospitalized for psychiatric treatment (Phillips et al. 1994).

Patients with BDD also have markedly poor quality of life. In a study that used the Medical Outcomes Study 36-Item Short-Form Health Survey (SF-36), BDD outpatients ($N = 62$) scored notably worse in all mental health domains than norms for the general U.S. population and for patients with depression, diabetes, or a recent myocardial infarction (Phillips 2000c). More severe BDD symptoms were associated with poorer mental health–related quality of life.

In one series, nearly 30% of patients with BDD had attempted suicide (Phillips et al. 1994). In a study of dermatological patients who committed suicide, most patients had acne or BDD (Cotterill and Cunliffe 1997).

Course

Data have consistently indicated that BDD usually begins during adolescence, with one series reporting a mean age at onset of 16 years and a mode of 13 (Phillips and Diaz 1997). Case studies and retrospective data indicate that BDD usually persists for years, if not decades, and tends to be unremitting, sometimes worsening over time (Phillips 1991). In a retrospective follow-up chart-review study of patients treated for BDD, a substantial percentage attained partial remission, but only a minority achieved and maintained full remission (Phillips et al. 1999).

Gender Similarities and Differences

Two studies that examined gender-related aspects of BDD found that the clinical features of the disorder appear to be similar in men and women. One of these studies ($N = 188$) found, however, that women were more likely than men to focus on their hips and weight, camouflage with makeup and pick their skin, and have comorbid bulimia nervosa (Phillips and Diaz 1997). In addition, the study found that men were more likely to be unmarried; be preoccupied with body build, genitals, and hair thinning; use a hat for camouflage; and have alcohol abuse or dependence. In the other study ($N = 58$), women were more likely to focus on their breasts and legs, check mirrors and camouflage, and have bulimia, panic disorder, and generalized anxiety disorder; men were more likely to focus on their genitals, height, and excessive body hair, and have bipolar disorder (Perugi et al. 1997a).

Muscle dysmorphia, in which a patient is preoccupied with the belief that he or she is too small and inadequate in muscularity, is a form of BDD that is far more common in men than in women (Pope et al. 1997), probably reflecting societal pressures for men to be muscular (Pope et al. 2000). This form of BDD is associated with typical BDD-related behaviors, such as camouflaging with clothing (to hide one's body or make it appear larger), mirror checking, and reassurance seeking, as well as compulsive working out (e.g., lifting weights) and use of dietary supplements. Some men with muscle dysmorphia use potentially dangerous anabolic steroids. This form of BDD usually interferes with social and occupational functioning and may lead to physical injury from excessive exercise.

BDD in Children and Adolescents

BDD usually begins during the early teenage years (Albertini and Phillips 1999). The clinical features of BDD in this age group appear to be similar to those in adults. In the largest published series of children and adolescents with BDD ($N = 33$), 95% had experienced social impairment and 87% had experienced academic impairment because of BDD, as evidenced, for example, by their avoidance of dating and other peer activities, stopping of athletic activities, and lateness to or absence from school (Albertini and Phillips 1999). Sixty-seven percent of patients had experienced suicidal ideation, 21% had attempted suicide, and 38% had engaged in violent behavior as a result of BDD. In addition, 39% of patients had been hospitalized for psychiatric treatment. These findings indicate that BDD can cause considerable morbidity in children and adolescents.

Cross-Cultural Aspects

Case reports and series from around the world suggest that the clinical features of BDD are similar across cultures, with culture producing nuances on a basically invariant, or universal, expression of BDD (Phillips 1996a).

Koro, a culture-related syndrome that may be related to BDD, occurs primarily in Southeast Asia. It is characterized by a preoccupation that the penis (labia, nipples, or breasts in women) is shrinking or retracting and will disappear into the abdomen, resulting in death (Chowdhury 1996). Although *koro* has similarities to BDD, it differs from BDD by its usually brief duration, different associated features (e.g., fear of death), response to reassurance, and occasional occurrence as an epidemic.

Case Study

Ms. A was an attractive 27-year-old single white female who presented with a chief complaint of "I look deformed." She had been convinced since she was a child that she was ugly, and her mother reported that she had "constantly been in the mirror" since she was a toddler. Ms. A was obsessed with many aspects of her appearance, including her "crooked" ears, "ugly" eyes, "broken out" skin, "huge" nose, and "bushy" facial hair. She estimated that she thought about her appearance for 16 hours a day and checked mirrors for 5 hours a day. She compulsively compared herself with other people, repeatedly sought reassurance about her appearance from her boyfriend and young son, applied and reapplied makeup for hours a day, excessively washed her face, covered her face with her hand, and tweezed and cut her facial hair. As a result of her appearance concerns, she had dropped out of high school and then college. She avoided friends and most social interactions. Ms. A felt chronically suicidal and had attempted suicide twice because, as she stated, "I'm too ugly to go on living."

Etiology and Pathophysiology

BDD's etiopathology is likely multifactorial, with neurobiological, evolutionary, sociocultural, and psychological factors playing a role. Family history data suggest that BDD is familial (K. A. Phillips, unpublished data). Neuropsychological studies indicate that the pathogenesis of BDD may involve executive dysfunction, implicating frontal-striatal pathology (Deckersbach et al. 2000; Hanes 1998). Rauch et al. (1998) hypothesized that BDD may involve dysfunction of the orbitofrontal system or the orbitofrontal-amygdalar axis, similar to OCD. Studies of this hypothesis are needed, as is investigation of the temporal and occipital lobes, which process facial images and, along with the parietal lobes, are involved in neurological disorders involving disturbed body image. Treatment data provide only indirect evidence about etiology but suggest a role for serotonin; antagonism of the serotonin system can worsen BDD symptoms.

In a study that used the Parental Bonding Instrument, BDD patients reported poorer parental care scores than published norms (Phillips et al. 1996b). It seems plausible that frequent criticism of or teasing about one's appearance could be a risk factor for BDD, but potential risk factors such as this have not been studied.

Relationship With Other Disorders

The paucity of studies comparing BDD with other disorders limits conclusions about their relationships. Most important, until the etiopathology of BDD and possibly related disorders is elucidated, the exact nature of their relationships will remain unknown.

The etiology and pathophysiology of these disorders are likely to be multifactorial and complex, involving both genetic (most likely, multiple genes of small effect) and environmental factors. It is likely that some of these disorders' pathogenic factors will be shown to overlap and others will be found to be distinct. Further complicating this issue is that BDD and related disorders are probably heterogeneous disorders.

Obsessive-Compulsive Disorder

BDD has many similarities to OCD, most notably prominent obsessions and repetitive behaviors. BDD has been considered to be an obsessive-compulsive spectrum disorder (Hollander 1993; McElroy et al. 1994), and it is probably more closely related to OCD than to the somatoform disorders with which it is classified. In a study that compared BDD and OCD, the disorders were similar in terms of sex ratio, illness severity, course of illness, and comorbidity (Phillips et al. 1998b). In addition, two neuropsychological studies found that BDD patients had deficits similar to those reported for OCD (Deckersbach et al. 2000; Hanes 1998), although BDD and OCD patients were directly compared in only one of the studies (Hanes 1998). However, the study comparing OCD and BDD found that BDD patients were less likely to be married, had poorer insight, and were more likely to have had suicidal ideation or made a suicide attempt because of their disorder (Phillips et al. 1998b). They also had earlier onset of major depression and higher lifetime rates of major depression, social phobia, and psychotic disorder diagnoses.

Although BDD's treatment response appears to be similar to that of OCD, BDD's response to serotonin reuptake inhibitor (SRI) augmentation appears to be different from that of OCD (Phillips et al. 2000a), and BDD may not respond as well as OCD to behavioral treatment without a cognitive component. Clinical observations suggest that BDD is more often characterized by shame, embarrassment, humiliation, low self-esteem, and rejection sensitivity and that BDD rituals are less likely to decrease anxiety (Phillips 1996a).

Clinical implications of these apparent differences include the following: 1) BDD patients need to be thoroughly assessed for depressive symptoms, suicidal ideation, and suicidal behavior; 2) the poorer insight of BDD patients may interfere with treatment compliance; and 3) BDD and OCD do not always respond to treatment concurrently (Phillips et al. 1998a); therefore, when they are comorbid, each disorder's symptoms should be identified, treated, and monitored.

Depression

BDD has also been postulated to be a symptom of depression (Carroll 1994) or related to depression (Phillips et al. 1994). BDD and depression are highly comorbid (Phillips and Diaz 1997), and both disorders are characterized by low self-esteem, rejection sensitivity, and feelings of unworthiness (Phillips et al. 1996a; Rosen and Ramirez 1998). However, BDD and depression have some notable differences (Phillips 1999), such as the presence of prominent obsessional preoccupations and repetitive behaviors in BDD. Many patients with depression focus less on their appearance, even neglecting it, rather than overfocusing on it. Patients with depression who dislike their appearance are unlikely to selectively and obsessionally focus on this aspect of themselves or spend hours a day performing compulsive appearance-related behaviors, such as mirror checking and reassurance seeking. Other apparent differences include the fact that BDD has a 1:1 sex ratio (Phillips and Diaz 1997), earlier age at onset (Phillips et al. 1993), and an often chronic course (Phillips et al. 1999). In addition, onset of BDD often precedes that of major depression, suggesting that BDD is not simply a symptom of depression (Phillips and Diaz 1997).

BDD and depression also appear to have a different treatment response, which has clinical implications. BDD appears to respond to SRIs but not to non-SRIs or electroconvulsive therapy (ECT), and treatment response time of BDD appears to be longer than that for depression (Phillips et al. 1998a). Higher SRI doses than are usually needed for treating depression often appear necessary for BDD (Phillips et al. 2000a). BDD and depression do not always respond to treatment concurrently (Phillips et al. 1998b). Unlike depression, BDD appears to respond to cognitive-behavioral therapy

(CBT) but not to other types of psychotherapy alone (Phillips et al. 1993).

Eating Disorders

Both BDD and eating disorders are characterized by disturbed body image, preoccupation with perceived appearance flaws, and performance of repetitive behaviors such as mirror checking and body measuring, and they have a similar age at onset. However, patients with eating disorders tend to dislike their weight and overall body size, whereas those with BDD dislike more specific body parts, often facial features (although this distinction is not always applicable). These disorders also differ in terms of sex ratio and are not as highly comorbid with each other as with many other disorders (Phillips and Diaz 1997). Family history and treatment data do not strongly support the hypothesis that these disorders are the same or closely related (Phillips et al. 1993).

Rosen and Ramirez (1998) found that BDD and eating disorders were characterized by similarly low levels of self-esteem and by equally severe body image symptoms and disturbance. However, patients with eating disorders reported more psychological symptoms on the Brief Symptom Inventory, and BDD patients had more diverse appearance concerns and more negative self-evaluation and avoidance of activities as a result of appearance concerns.

Delusional Versus Nondelusional BDD

A clinically important controversy is whether delusional BDD (a psychotic disorder) and nondelusional BDD (a somatoform disorder) are the same or different disorders. In DSM-IV, delusional and nondelusional BDD may be double coded so that patients who are delusional receive both diagnoses, reflecting clinical and empirical evidence that these conditions are the same disorder, spanning a spectrum of insight. Indeed, delusional and nondelusional BDD have more similarities than differences, although the delusional variant appears to be more severe (Phillips et al. 1994). Consistent with these findings, both delusional and nondelusional patients appear to respond to SRIs but not to antipsychotics alone.

Diagnosis

BDD is often difficult to diagnose because patients usually do not disclose their symptoms as a result of embarrassment and shame (Phillips 2000a). Unless BDD is specifically asked about, the diagnosis is usually missed (Phillips et al. 1996a; Zimmerman and Mattia 1998). Not diagnosing BDD is problematic because treatment may be unsuccessful and the patient may feel misunderstood and inadequately informed about the diagnosis and treatment options. BDD can be diagnosed with the following questions, which reflect DSM-IV diagnostic criteria:

- Are you concerned about your appearance in any way? If so, what is your concern?
- Does this concern preoccupy you? That is, do you think about it a lot and wish you could worry about it less?
- What effect has this preoccupation with your appearance had on your life? Has it significantly interfered with your social life, school work, job, other activities, or other aspects of your life?
- Have your appearance concerns caused you a lot of distress?
- Have your appearance concerns affected your family or friends?

Clues to the diagnosis include all of the BDD-related behaviors described previously, ideas or delusions of reference, the confining of oneself to the house, unnecessary surgical or dermatological treatment, depression, anxiety, panic attacks, social anxiety and self-consciousness, and suicidal ideation. BDD is often misdiagnosed as one of the following disorders:

- *Depression.* Depressive symptoms often coexist with BDD, which may lead to a diagnosis of depression but not BDD.
- *Social phobia or avoidant personality disorder.* Social anxiety is a common consequence of BDD, which may lead to a misdiagnosis of social phobia or avoidant personality disorder.
- *Agoraphobia.* BDD patients may be housebound, which may lead to a misdiagnosis of agoraphobia.

- *Panic disorder.* Panic attacks that occur when a BDD patient looks in the mirror or experiences referential thinking may lead to a misdiagnosis of panic disorder.
- *Trichotillomania.* Some patients remove their hair (e.g., facial hair) in an effort to improve their appearance, which may lead to a misdiagnosis of trichotillomania.
- *Schizophrenia or psychotic disorder not otherwise specified.* BDD patients are often delusional, which may lead to a misdiagnosis of schizophrenia or psychotic disorder not otherwise specified.

Treatment

In the psychiatric literature, BDD has been said to be "extremely difficult" to treat (Munro and Chmara 1982). As a noted dermatologist stated, "The author knows of no more difficult patients to treat than those with body dysmorphic disorder" (Cotterill 1996, p. 463). Despite this pessimism, emerging evidence suggests that two forms of treatment are often effective for this disorder: 1) pharmacotherapy with SRIs or selective SRIs (SSRIs) and 2) CBT.

Pharmacotherapy

SRIs often appear to be effective, and more effective than other medications, for treating BDD (Phillips 2000b). After several small case series reported response to SRIs (Brady et al. 1990; Hollander et al. 1989), data from a series of 30 patients indicated that 58% responded to SRIs, whereas only 5% responded to other medications (Phillips et al. 1993). This series was expanded to 130 patients (who received a total of 316 medications) for whom responses were assessed retrospectively (Phillips 1996c). The percentages of trials that resulted in improvement were 42% of 65 trials with an SRI; 30% of 23 trials with monoamine oxidase inhibitors (MAOIs), 15% of 48 trials with non-SRI tricyclics; 3% of trials with neuroleptics; 6% of trials with a variety of other medications (e.g., mood stabilizers); and 0% of trials with ECT.

In a series of 45 patients treated in the author's clinical practice, 43 (70%) of 61 SRI trials resulted in improvement (Phillips

1996c). The higher response rate to SRIs for the prospectively treated patients is likely attributable to the higher doses and longer treatment trials used. In a retrospective study of 50 patients, 35 SRI trials resulted in much improvement, whereas 18 non-SRI (i.e., tricyclic) trials led to no overall improvement in BDD symptoms (Hollander et al. 1994).

In a 16-week open-label study of fluvoxamine, 19 (63%) of 30 patients responded (mean dose = 238.3 ± 85.8 mg/day; mean time to response = 6.1 ± 3.7 weeks, range = 1 to 16 weeks) (Phillips et al. 1998a). In a 10-week open-label fluvoxamine study, 10 (67%) of 15 patients responded (Perugi et al. 1996). A controlled pharmacotherapy BDD trial—a double-blind crossover study of 40 patients (29 of whom were randomized)—found that clomipramine was more effective than desipramine (Hollander et al. 1999). At the end of the study's first phase, 65% of patients had responded to clomipramine and 35% had responded to desipramine. Response to medication usually results in improved functioning and decreased appearance-related preoccupations, distress, and behaviors.

Clinical experience suggests that all SRIs may be effective for BDD (Phillips et al. 2000b). In a clinical practice setting, discontinuation of an effective SRI led to relapse of BDD in 83% ($N = 31$) of cases. This finding suggests that long-term treatment is often needed. Clinical experience also suggests that SRI efficacy for BDD is usually sustained over time.

Several of the aforementioned studies assessed treatment response in patients who were delusional and found that these patients also responded to SRIs (Hollander et al. 1999; Phillips and McElroy 1993; Phillips et al. 1994, 1998b) and that delusionality often improved with SRI treatment (Phillips et al. 1998a). Delusions were likely to be a heterogeneous phenomenon (Garety 1998), with the delusions that can occur in OCD and putative obsessive-compulsive spectrum disorders (e.g., BDD, hypochondriasis, anorexia nervosa) differing from more "classic" delusions (e.g., those of schizophrenia and mood disorders) in terms of etiology, pathophysiology, and treatment response. It seems likely that only delusions characteristic of obsessive-compulsive spectrum disorders respond to SRIs alone.

The aforementioned studies found that other medications for BDD were less effective than SRIs. An important question is whether antipsychotics are effective as monotherapy for delusional BDD. The antipsychotic pimozide, in particular, has been said to be uniquely effective for treating monosymptomatic hypochondriacal psychosis, including delusional BDD (Munro and Chmara 1982). However, available data suggest that antipsychotics alone, including pimozide, are unlikely to be effective for delusional BDD (Phillips et al. 1994), although these data are largely retrospective and therefore limited. Case series and reports have suggested that ECT is generally ineffective for treating BDD (Phillips 2000b).

Because SRI response is often partial, augmentation strategies are of interest and importance. An open-label study (Phillips 1996b) and a study from a clinical practice setting (Phillips et al. 2000a) found that buspirone augmentation was effective, although in a minority of cases. In the open-label study, the mean time to response was 6.4 ± 1.7 weeks (range = 5 to 9 weeks) and the mean effective dose was 48.3 ± 14.7 mg/day (range = 30 to 60 mg/day). Several patients further improved with higher doses (70–90 mg/day). Combining clomipramine with an SSRI may also be effective, although clomipramine blood levels must be monitored (Phillips et al. 2000a). The addition of a neuroleptic is worth considering for patients who are delusional (Phillips et al. 2000a). Some patients with severe depressive symptoms may benefit from SRI augmentation with lithium or a stimulant, which may alleviate depressive symptoms and thereby improve the overall clinical picture (Phillips 2000b). Patients who do not respond to an SRI may respond to another SRI or venlafaxine (Phillips et al. 2000a). If none of these strategies is effective, an MAOI may be worth trying.

Although these data suggest that SRIs are selectively effective for BDD, controlled treatment trials—in particular, placebo-controlled trials—are needed to confirm these findings. Relatively high SRI doses often appear necessary to effectively treat BDD, but dose finding studies are needed to determine optimal SRI doses. It appears that treatment response often requires 10–12 weeks and that long-term treatment is often needed (Phillips et al. 1998a);

however, further investigation is needed to help determine the minimal duration of an adequate treatment trial and optimal treatment duration. Finally, studies that compare different SRIs and studies of augmentation, as well as continuation, maintenance, and discontinuation studies, are needed.

Cognitive-Behavioral Therapy

CBT is a promising approach for treating BDD. Early case reports indicated a successful outcome with exposure therapy (Marks and Mishan 1988; Schmidt and Harrington 1995), audiovisual self-confrontation (Klages and Hartwich 1982), systematic desensitization (Munjack 1978), and cognitive plus behavioral techniques (Cromarty and Marks 1995; Gomez-Perez et al. 1994; Newell and Schrubb 1994). Studies using exposure (e.g., exposing the perceived defect in social situations and preventing avoidance behaviors), response prevention (e.g., helping the patient avoid compulsive behaviors, such as mirror checking), and cognitive restructuring have found these approaches to be effective for a majority of patients. In a report of 5 patients, 4 improved using these techniques in 90-minute sessions 1 or 5 days per week (with the total number of sessions ranging from 12 to 48) (Neziroglu and Yaryura-Tobias 1993). Techniques included covering or removing mirrors, limiting grooming time, stopping use of makeup, and having patients sit in crowded waiting rooms. In an open series of 13 patients treated with group CBT, BDD significantly improved in twelve 90-minute group sessions (Wilhelm et al. 1999). In a study of 10 patients who participated in an intensive behavioral therapy program, including a 6-month maintenance program, improvement was maintained for up to 2 years (McKay 1999).

Two studies used a waiting-list control design. In a study of eight weekly 2-hour sessions of group CBT, cognitive techniques plus exposure and response prevention were effective for 27 (77%) of 35 women, with patients in the CBT group improving more than those in the no-treatment waiting-list control group (Rosen et al. 1995). However, patients appeared to have relatively mild BDD, and many seemed to be in a "diagnostic gray zone" between BDD and eating disorders. In a pilot study of 19 patients, there was significantly greater improvement among patients who participated in group CBT than among patients in a no-treatment waiting-list control group, with the symptoms of 7 (77%) of 9 patients no longer meeting criteria for BDD (Veale et al. 1996b). It is unclear whether exposure and response prevention alone are effective for treating BDD. Some studies suggest that it is effective (McKay et al. 1997), whereas others indicate that it is not and suggest that cognitive restructuring is a necessary component of treatment (Campisi 1995), perhaps because of the poor insight and depression characteristic of BDD.

Data on CBT, although promising, are from clinical series and studies using a waiting-list control design, which does not control for therapist attention and other nonspecific treatment factors. Psychotherapy studies using an attention control group or an alternative treatment are needed. Also requiring empirical investigation are questions about whether a cognitive component is necessary; whether CBT alone is effective for patients who are severely depressed, suicidal, and delusional; and whether booster sessions are needed. Further study is needed to determine the minimum number of required sessions and session frequency. In published studies, the number of treatment sessions varied from twelve 90-minute sessions (Wilhelm et al. 1999) to forty-eight 90-minute sessions (Neziroglu and Yaryura-Tobias 1993), whereas in clinical settings, far fewer sessions may be available because of insurance limitations.

Insight-Oriented and Supportive Psychotherapy

Available data suggest that BDD symptoms—especially severe symptoms—are unlikely to significantly improve with insight-oriented or supportive psychotherapy alone (Phillips et al. 1993). However, these treatments may be effective for other disorders or problems the patient may have, and patients benefit from the support they receive in coping with their illness, whether provided as more formal supportive psychotherapy or as part of CBT or medication treatment.

Surgery and Nonpsychiatric Medical Treatment

A notable aspect of BDD—from a clinical, public health, and cost perspective—is the high rate of surgical (Fukuda 1977), dermatological (Cotterill 1996), dental (Phillips et al. 1993), and other medical treatment (Phillips et al. 1993) sought and received. A majority of patients seen in a psychiatric setting have received such treatment, most often dermatological treatment and surgery (Phillips et al. 1994). The dermatological literature notes that BDD patients request extensive work-ups, consult numerous physicians, and pressure dermatologists to prescribe unsuitable and ineffective treatments (Cotterill 1996).

These treatments usually appear to be ineffective and may even worsen appearance concerns (Andreasen and Bardach 1977; Phillips and Diaz 1997). The dermatological and surgical literature indicates that the outcome of such treatments is often poor (Cotterill 1996; Fukuda 1977). Occasionally, dissatisfied patients commit suicide or are violent toward the treating physician, even threatening or committing murder (Phillips 1991). Some patients perform their own surgery, as did one man who cut his nose open and tried to replace his own cartilage with chicken cartilage (Phillips 1996a).

Treatment Strategies

On the basis of available data and the author's clinical experience, the following treatment strategies are recommended (Phillips 2000a):

- Target BDD symptoms in treatment. Ignoring BDD symptoms and focusing treatment on depression only, for example, may be unsuccessful.
- Use an SRI as a first-line approach, even for patients who are delusional. Although most published data are on fluvoxamine and clomipramine, other SRIs and venlafaxine appear to be effective.
- Use the maximum SRI dose recommended or tolerated if lower doses are ineffective. BDD appears to often require SRI doses higher than those typically used for treating depression (Phillips et al. 2000a).

- Treat the patient for 12–16 weeks before assessing SRI response (Phillips et al. 1998a).
- Continue an effective SRI for at least 1 year, because relapse appears likely with discontinuation (Phillips et al. 2000a). Severely ill patients may require lifelong treatment.
- Although all SRIs appear to be effective, one may be more effective than another for an individual patient; if one SRI fails, another should be tried, because some patients respond to the third, fourth, or fifth SRI tried (Phillips et al. 2000a).
- Avoid using antipsychotics as monotherapy for BDD, even for patients who are delusional.
- Antipsychotic augmentation of an SRI is a reasonable approach for delusional patients who do not respond to an SRI or for severely ill delusional patients as initial treatment in combination with an SRI; clinical experience suggests that atypical antipsychotics may be more effective than typical antipsychotics and are likely to be better tolerated (Phillips 2000a).
- Consider using CBT as a first-line approach, especially for patients with milder BDD without significant comorbidity requiring pharmacotherapy.
- Use more intensive CBT treatment (e.g., frequent sessions, use of homework) rather than less intensive treatment.
- Use a cognitive component in addition to exposure and response prevention.
- Consider maintenance/booster sessions for patients with more severe BDD following treatment to prevent relapse.
- For patients with severe BDD, especially patients who are very depressed or suicidal, use CBT only in combination with medication, because sicker patients may not be able to tolerate or participate in CBT. Partial response to medication can make CBT possible.
- Avoid using supportive or insight-oriented psychotherapy as the only treatment, especially for patients whose BDD is more severe, but consider adding supportive psychotherapy to an SRI and/or CBT for certain patients, including patients who 1) have significant life stressors, 2) have a personality disorder requiring psychotherapy, 3) need couples or family therapy, 4) comply poorly with treatment, or 5) have severe BDD symp-

toms and need additional monitoring and support.

- Encourage patients to avoid surgery and other nonpsychiatric medical treatment; however, patients who pick their skin may need dermatological treatment in combination with psychiatric treatment.
- Consider psychoeducation as an important aspect of treatment.
- Consider involving family members in the treatment when appropriate, because they may provide support to the patient and facilitate treatment.
- For treatment-resistant patients, 1) ensure that SRI or CBT treatment is adequate (a higher SRI dose, more frequent CBT sessions, or a longer treatment trial may be effective); 2) consider adding CBT to an SRI or vice versa; and 3) consider SRI pharmacologic augmentation.

Conclusion

Research on BDD has dramatically increased in recent years, and much has been learned about its clinical features and treatment. Although BDD is often difficult to treat, available treatment strategies are very promising. Given how distressing BDD can be, and the profound disability it can cause, it is important for clinicians to screen patients for this disorder, keeping in mind that patients typically do not reveal their symptoms unless specifically asked about them. Until more is known about BDD's relationship with other disorders, such as OCD and depression, it is important that BDD be differentiated from other disorders and targeted during treatment.

References

Albertini RS, Phillips KA: Thirty-three cases of body dysmorphic disorder in children and adolescents. J Am Acad Child Adolesc Psychiatry 38:453–459, 1999

American Psychiatric Association: Diagnostic and Statistical Manual of Mental Disorders, 3rd Edition. Washington, DC, American Psychiatric Association, 1980

American Psychiatric Association: Diagnostic and Statistical Manual of
   Mental Disorders, 3rd Edition, Revised. Washington, DC, American
   Psychiatric Association, 1987

American Psychiatric Association: Diagnostic and Statistical Manual of
   Mental Disorders, 4th Edition. Washington, DC, American Psychiatric Association, 1994

Andreasen NC, Bardach J: Dysmorphophobia: symptom or disease?
   Am J Psychiatry 134:673–675, 1977

Biby EL: The relationship between body dysmorphic disorder and
   depression, self-esteem, somatization, and obsessive-compulsive
   disorder. J Clin Psychol 54:489–499, 1998

Bienvenu OJ, Samuels JF, Riddle MA, et al: The relationship of obsessive-compulsive disorder to possible spectrum disorders: results
   from a family study. Biol Psychiatry 48:287–293, 2000

Brady KT, Austin L, Lydiard RB: Body dysmorphic disorder: the relationship to obsessive-compulsive disorder. J Nerv Ment Dis 178:538–
   540, 1990

Brawman-Mintzer O, Lydiard RB, Phillips KA, et al: Body dysmorphic
   disorder in patients with anxiety disorders and major depression: a
   comorbidity study. Am J Psychiatry 152:1665–1667, 1995

Campisi T: Cognitive therapy in the treatment of body dysmorphic disorder. Unpublished doctoral dissertation, Hofstra University, Great
   Neck, New York, 1995

Carroll BJ: Response of major depression with psychosis and body dysmorphic disorder to ECT (letter). Am J Psychiatry 151:288–289, 1994

Chowdhury AN: The definition and classification of koro. Cult Med
   Psychiatry 20:41–65, 1996

Cotterill JA: Body dysmorphic disorder. Dermatol Clin 14:457–463, 1996

Cotterill JA, Cunliffe WJ: Suicide in dermatological patients. Br J Dermatol 137:246–250, 1997

Cromarty P, Marks I: Does rational role-play enhance the outcome of
   exposure therapy in dysmorphophobia? A case study. Br J Psychiatry
   167:399–402, 1995

Deckersbach T, Savage CR, Phillips KA, et al: Characteristics of memory
   dysfunction in body dysmorphic disorder. J Int Neuropsychol Soc 6:
   673–681, 2000

DeMarco LM, Li LC, Phillips KA, et al: Perceived stress in body dysmorphic disorder. J Nerv Ment Dis 186:724–726, 1998

Faravelli C, Salvatori S, Galassi F, et al: Epidemiology of somatoform
   disorders: a community survey in Florence. Soc Psychiatry Psychiatr
   Epidemiol 32:24–29, 1997

Fukuda O: Statistical analysis of dysmorphophobia in out-patient clinic. Japanese Journal of Plastic and Reconstructive Surgery 20:569–577, 1977

Garety PA: Insight and delusions, in Insight and Psychosis. Edited by Amador XF, David AS. New York, Oxford University Press, 1998, pp 66–77

Gomez-Perez JC, Marks IM, Gutierrez-Fisac JL: Dysmorphophobia: clinical features and outcome with behavior therapy. European Psychiatry 9:229–235, 1994

Hanes KR: Neuropsychological performance in body dysmorphic disorder. J Int Neuropsychol Soc 4:167–171, 1998

Hardy GE: Body image disturbance in dysmorphophobia. Br J Psychiatry 141:181–185, 1982

Hollander E: Introduction, in Obsessive-Compulsive Related Disorders. Edited by Hollander E. Washington, DC, American Psychiatric Press, 1993, pp 1–16

Hollander E, Liebowitz MR, Winchel R, et al: Treatment of body-dysmorphic disorder with serotonin reuptake blockers. Am J Psychiatry 146:768–770, 1989

Hollander E, Cohen LJ, Simeon D: Body dysmorphic disorder. Psychiatric Annals 23:359–364, 1993

Hollander E, Cohen L, Simeon D, et al: Fluvoxamine treatment of body dysmorphic disorder (letter). J Clin Psychopharmacol 14:75–77, 1994

Hollander E, Allen A, Kwon J, et al: Clomipramine vs desipramine crossover trial in body dysmorphic disorder: selective efficacy of a serotonin reuptake inhibitor in imagined ugliness. Arch Gen Psychiatry 56:1033–1039, 1999

Ishigooka J, Iwao M, Suzuki M, et al: Demographic features of patients seeking cosmetic surgery. Psychiatry Clin Neurosci 52:283–287, 1998

Janet P: Les Obsessions et la Psychasthenie. Paris, Felix Alcan, 1903

Jerome L: Body size estimation in characterizing dysmorphic symptoms in patients with body dysmorphic disorder (letter). Am J Psychiatry 36:620, 1991

Klages W, Hartwich P: Die clowndysmorphophobie. Psychother Psychosom Med Psychol 32:183–187, 1982

Kraepelin E: Psychiatrie, 8th Edition. Leipzig, JA Barth, 1909–1915

Ladee GA: Hypochondriacal Syndromes. Amsterdam, Elsevier, 1966

Marks I, Mishan J: Dysmorphophobic avoidance with disturbed bodily perception: a pilot study of exposure therapy. Br J Psychiatry 152:674–678, 1988

Mayville S, Katz RC, Gipson MT, et al: Assessing the prevalence of body dysmorphic disorder in an ethnically diverse group of adolescents. Journal of Child and Family Studies 8:357–362, 1999

McElroy SL, Phillips KA, Keck PE Jr: Obsessive compulsive spectrum disorder. J Clin Psychiatry 55(suppl 10):33–51, 1994

McKay D. Two-year follow-up of behavioral treatment and maintenance for body dysmorphic disorder. Behav Modif 23:620–629, 1999

McKay D, Todaro J, Neziroglu F, et al: Body dysmorphic disorder: a preliminary evaluation of treatment and maintenance using exposure with response prevention. Behav Res Ther 35:67–70, 1997

Morselli E: Sulla dismorfofobia e sulla tafefobia. Bolletinno della R accademia di Genova, 6:110–119, 1891

Munjack DJ: The behavioral treatment of dysmorphophobia. J Behav Ther Exp Psychiatry 9:53–56, 1978

Munro A, Chmara J: Monosymptomatic hypochondriacal psychosis: a diagnostic checklist based on 50 cases of the disorder. Can J Psychiatry 27:374–376, 1982

Newell R, Schrubb S: Attitude change and behaviour therapy in body dysmorphic disorder: two case reports. Behavioural and Cognitive Psychotherapy 22:163–169, 1994

Neziroglu FA, Yaryura-Tobias JA: Exposure, response prevention, and cognitive therapy in the treatment of body dysmorphic disorder. Behavior Therapy 24:431–438, 1993

Neziroglu F, McKay D, Todaro J, et al: Effect of cognitive behavior therapy on persons with body dysmorphic disorder and comorbid axis II diagnoses. Behavior Therapy 27:67–77, 1996

O'Sullivan RL, Phillips KA, Keuthen NJ, et al: Near-fatal skin picking from delusional body dysmorphic disorder responsive to fluvoxamine. Psychosomatics 40:79–81, 1999

Perugi G, Giannotti D, Di Vaio S, et al: Fluvoxamine in the treatment of body dysmorphic disorder (dysmorphophobia). Int Clin Psychopharmacol 11:247–254, 1996

Perugi G, Akiskal HS, Giannotti D, et al: Gender-related differences in body dysmorphic disorder (dysmorphophobia). J Nerv Ment Dis 185:578–582, 1997

Perugi G, Akiskal HS, Lattanzi L, et al: The high prevalence of "soft" bipolar (II) features in atypical depression. Compr Psychiatry 39:63–71, 1998

Phillips KA: Body dysmorphic disorder: the distress of imagined ugliness. Am J Psychiatry 148:1138–1149, 1991

Phillips KA: The Broken Mirror: Recognizing and Treating Body Dysmorphic Disorder. New York, Oxford University Press, 1996a

Phillips KA: An open study of buspirone augmentation of serotonin-reuptake inhibitors in body dysmorphic disorder. Psychopharmacol Bull 32:175–180, 1996b

Phillips KA: Pharmacologic treatment of body dysmorphic disorder. Psychopharmacol Bull 32:597–605, 1996c

Phillips KA: Body dysmorphic disorder and depression: theoretical considerations and treatment strategies. Psychiatr Q 70:313–331, 1999

Phillips KA. Body dysmorphic disorder: diagnostic controversies and treatment challenges. Bull Menninger Clin 64:18–35, 2000a

Phillips KA: Pharmacologic treatment of body dysmorphic disorder: a review of empirical data and a proposed treatment algorithm. Psychiatr Clin North Am 7:59–82, 2000b

Phillips KA: Quality of life for patients with body dysmorphic disorder. J Nerv Ment Dis 188:170–175, 2000c

Phillips KA, Diaz SF: Gender differences in body dysmorphic disorder. J Nerv Ment Dis 185:570–577, 1997

Phillips KA, McElroy SL: Insight, overvalued ideation, and delusional thinking in body dysmorphic disorder: theoretical and treatment implications. J Nerv Ment Dis 181:699–702, 1993

Phillips KA, McElroy SL: Personality disorders and traits in patients with body dysmorphic disorder. Compr Psychiatry 41:229–236, 2000

Phillips KA, Taub SL: Skin picking as a symptom of body dysmorphic disorder. Psychopharmacol Bull 31:279–288, 1995

Phillips KA, McElroy SL, Keck PE Jr, et al: Body dysmorphic disorder: 30 cases of imagined ugliness. Am J Psychiatry 150:302–308, 1993

Phillips KA, McElroy SL, Keck PE Jr: A comparison of delusional and nondelusional body dysmorphic disorder in 100 cases. Psychopharmacol Bull 30:179–186, 1994

Phillips KA, Nierenberg AA, Brendel G, et al: Prevalence and clinical features of body dysmorphic disorder in atypical major depression. J Nerv Ment Dis 184:125–129, 1996a

Phillips KA, Steketee G, Shapiro L: Parental bonding in OCD and body dysmorphic disorder, in 1996 New Research Program and Abstracts, American Psychiatric Association 149th Annual Meeting, New York, May 4–9, 1996. Washington, DC, American Psychiatric Association, 1996b, p 261

Phillips KA, Dwight MM, McElroy SL: Efficacy and safety of fluvoxamine in body dysmorphic disorder. J Clin Psychiatry 59:165–171, 1998a

Phillips KA, Gunderson CG, Mallya G, et al: A comparison study of body dysmorphic disorder and obsessive-compulsive disorder. J Clin Psychiatry 59:568–575, 1998b

Phillips KA, Grant J, Albertini RS, et al: Retrospective follow-up study of body dysmorphic disorder, in 1999 New Research Program and Abstracts, American Psychiatric Association 152nd Annual Meeting, Washington, DC, May 15–20, 1999. Washington, DC, American Psychiatric Association, 1999, p 151

Phillips KA, Albertini RS, Khan AA, et al: Effectiveness of pharmacotherapy for body dysmorphic disorder: a chart-review study, in New Clinical Drug Evaluation Unit (NCDEU) 40th Annual Meeting: Abstracts of Posters and Presentations. Bethesda, MD, National Institute of Mental Health, 2000a, p 180

Phillips KA, Dufresne RG Jr, Wilkel C, et al: Rate of body dysmorphic disorder in dermatology patients. J Am Acad Dermatol 42:436–441, 2000b

Piggott TA, L'Heureux F, Dubbert B, et al: Obsessive compulsive disorder: comorbid conditions. J Clin Psychiatry 55(no 10, suppl):15–27, 1994

Pope HG Jr, Gruber AJ, Choi P, et al: Muscle dysmorphia. An underrecognized form of body dysmorphic disorder. Psychosomatics 38:548–557, 1997

Pope HG, Phillips KA, Olivardia R: The Adonis Complex: The Secret Crisis of Male Body Obsession. New York, Free Press, 2000

Rauch SL, Whalen PJ, Dougherty D: Neurobiologic models of obsessive-compulsive disorder, in Obsessive-Compulsive Disorders: Practical Management, 3rd Edition. Edited by Jenike MA, Baer L, Minichiello WE. St Louis, CV Mosby, 1998, pp 222–253

Rosen JC, Ramirez E: A comparison of eating disorders and body dysmorphic disorder on body image and psychological adjustment. J Psychosom Res 44:441–449, 1998

Rosen JC, Reiter J, Orosan P: Cognitive-behavioral body image therapy for body dysmorphic disorder. J Consult Clin Psychol 63:263–269, 1995

Sarwer DB, Wadden TA, Pertschuk MJ, et al: Body image dissatisfaction and body dysmorphic disorder in 100 cosmetic surgery patients. Plast Reconstr Surg 101:1644–1649, 1998a

Sarwer DB, Whitaker LA, Pertschuk MJ, et al: Body image concerns of reconstructive surgery patients: an underrecognized problem. Ann Plast Surg 40:403–407, 1998b

Schmidt NB, Harrington P: Cognitive-behavioral treatment of body dysmorphic disorder: a case report. J Behav Ther Exp Psychiatry 26: 161–167, 1995

Simeon D, Hollander E, Stein DJ, et al: Body dysmorphic disorder in the DSM-IV field trial for obsessive-compulsive disorder. Am J Psychiatry 152:1207–1209, 1995

Soriano JL, O'Sullivan RL, Baer L, et al: Trichotillomania and self-esteem: a survey of 62 female hair pullers. J Clin Psychiatry 57:77–82, 1996

Thomas CS, Goldberg DP: Appearance, body image and distress in facial dysmorphophobia. Acta Psychiatr Scand 92:231–236, 1995

Veale D, Boocock A, Gournay K, et al: Body dysmorphic disorder. A survey of fifty cases. Br J Psychiatry 169:196–201, 1996a

Veale D, Gournay K, Dryden W, et al: Body dysmorphic disorder: a cognitive behavioural model and pilot randomised controlled trial. Behav Res Ther 34:717–729, 1996b

Wilhelm S, Otto MW, Zucker BG, et al: Prevalence of body dysmorphic disorder in patients with anxiety disorders. J Anxiety Disord 11:499–502, 1997

Wilhelm S, Otto MW, Lohr B, et al: Cognitive behavior group therapy for body dysmorphic disorder: a case series. Behav Res Ther 37:71–75, 1999

Zimmerman M, Mattia JI: Body dysmorphic disorder in psychiatric outpatients: recognition, prevalence, comorbidity, demographic, and clinical correlates. Compr Psychiatry 39:265–270, 1998

Chapter 4

Conversion Disorder

José R. Maldonado, M.D.
David Spiegel, M.D.

Dsm-I (American Psychiatric Association 1952) described conversion reactions as functional symptoms in organs or body parts, usually under voluntary control, resulting from conversion of impulses causing anxiety from psychological to somatic form. In DSM-II (American Psychiatric Association 1968), conversion (then known as hysterical neurosis, conversion type) was considered an involuntary psychogenic loss of function in which symbolism of the symptom, hysterical personality, secondary gain, and the presence of "la belle indifférence" were of diagnostic importance. However, after a review of the literature, Lazare (1981) concluded that these descriptions had no diagnostic validity.

DSM-III (American Psychiatric Association 1980) specified that conversion disorder consists of a loss or alteration in physical functioning that cannot be explained by a medical condition. It further specified that the disorder is *not* under voluntary control and that psychological factors are etiologically related to the onset of the symptoms or deficits.

DSM-IV (American Psychiatric Association 1994) established six criteria for the diagnosis of conversion disorder, and these criteria remain unchanged in DSM-IV-TR (American Psychiatric Association 2000) (Table 4–1). The essential diagnostic feature (Criterion A) is the presence of "symptoms or deficits affecting voluntary motor or sensory function that suggest a neurological or other general medical condition." Although this criterion was used in DSM-I and DSM-II, it was broadened in DSM-III to include symptoms involving "any loss of, or alteration in, physical functioning suggesting a physical disorder."

Table 4–1. DSM-IV-TR diagnostic criteria for conversion disorder

A. One or more symptoms or deficits affecting voluntary motor or sensory function that suggest a neurological or other general medical condition.

B. Psychological factors are judged to be associated with the symptom or deficit because the initiation or exacerbation of the symptom or deficit is preceded by conflicts or other stressors.

C. The symptom or deficit is not intentionally produced or feigned (as in factitious disorder or malingering).

D. The symptom or deficit cannot, after appropriate investigation, be fully explained by a general medical condition, or by the direct effects of a substance, or as a culturally sanctioned behavior or experience.

E. The symptom or deficit causes clinically significant distress or impairment in social, occupational, or other important areas of functioning or warrants medical evaluation.

F. The symptom or deficit is not limited to pain or sexual dysfunction, does not occur exclusively during the course of somatization disorder, and is not better accounted for by another mental disorder.

Specify type of symptom or deficit:

With Motor Symptom or Deficit
With Sensory Symptom or Deficit
With Seizures or Convulsions
With Mixed Presentation

Source. Reprinted with permission from American Psychiatric Association: *Diagnostic and Statistical Manual of Mental Disorders,* 4th Edition, Text Revision. Washington, DC, American Psychiatric Association, 2000, p. 498. Copyright 2000, American Psychiatric Association.

There has been controversy regarding whether conversion disorder should be included among the somatoform or dissociative disorders. It has remained with the somatoform disorders to maintain the uniformity of "diagnoses that suggest physical disorders." Nevertheless, ICD-10 calls the condition "dissociative (conversion) disorders," consistent with historical psychopathological theories regarding the etiological and mechanistic views of hysteria and conversion (World Health Organization 1992).

DSM-IV-TR Criterion B establishes that psychological factors are associated with the initiation and maintenance of the symptoms or deficits. Criterion C rules out intentional (feigned) symptom production, as in the case of factitious disorder or malingering. Criterion D establishes that a neurological or other general medical cause needs to be ruled out. It also dictates that culturally sanctioned behavior or experiences (e.g., possession syndrome) may not be diagnosed as a conversion disorder. Criterion E establishes the clinical significance of the symptoms as evidenced by the presence of significant distress, social or occupational impairment, or the pursuit of medical evaluation and treatment. Finally, Criterion F differentiates conversion disorder from pain disorder, sexual dysfunction, somatization disorder, and other Axis I diagnoses.

Clinical Subtypes

Historically, the most common conversion symptoms were paralysis, somnambulism, convulsive attacks, and afflictions of the senses, as in blindness and mutism (Janet 1925). Nevertheless, conversion disorder may mimic many neurological, medical, and psychiatric disorders. DSM-IV-TR recognizes four conversion disorder subtypes based on the nature of the presenting symptoms. These subtypes include conversion presenting with primarily motor symptoms or deficits, sensory symptoms or deficits, seizures (e.g., pseudoseizures), and mixed presentations of these symptoms.

Motor Symptoms or Deficits

Abnormalities in the musculoskeletal system may involve tremors, usually affecting the limbs, head, and trunk. Tremors tend to be coarse and not intentional, with the tendency to worsen when attention is directed to them. Occasionally, complex and stereotyped choreiform tics and jerks may occur. Muscle spasms, usually associated with pseudoseizures and sometimes affecting the entire body, may be seen, especially in mixed presentations (Janet 1907, 1920, 1925; Lazare 1978; Ljundberg 1957; Roy 1980).

Some dramatic motor presentations were described by Charcot (1889) and Janet (1907) and can be seen today. These include catatonic-like postures (*attitudes passionelles*); gait disturbance with staggering and stumbling; abnormal trunk movements, with wobbling from the hips and clutching at the air and walls for support (*astasia-abasia*); pareses; and paralyses.

Because of the psychological nature of the deficit, the loss of motor function reflects the patient's perception of neurological function rather than neural innervation. Thus, on occasion dissociation of function is seen. This phenomenon involves the apparent lack of function of an organ or limb for certain purposes, such as writing, but no apparent difficulties in performing other tasks or functions with the same organ or limb, such as scratching.

In an attempt to maintain the deficit, it is common for a patient to have a tonic contracture of antagonistic muscles around a joint, thus immobilizing that extremity (Fallik and Sigal 1971; Farley et al. 1968; Guze and Perley 1963; Janet 1907; Miller 1986; Pilowsky 1969; Reismann and Singh 1978). On passive examination of the affected extremity, the clinician will find a contraction in the patient's musculature that is opposite in direction, but proportional in strength, to that applied by the clinician. Other motor dysfunctions may involve difficulty swallowing, creating aphagia or "globus hystericus," or paresis of the muscles of phonation, causing partial or total aphonia (Deary et al. 1989; Leigh and Riley 1988; Puhakka and Kirveskari 1988; Wilson et al. 1988, 1991).

Sensory Symptoms or Deficits

Conversion disorder can present with alterations of almost any sensory modality. The distribution of the disturbance is inconsistent with anatomical sensory innervation and sometimes is inconsistent over time. In the visual system, blindness, changes (e.g., double vision, blurred vision) or constriction of the visual fields, "tunnel" or "gun barrel" vision (e.g., peripheral blindness with preservation of central vision), and visual hallucinations have been described (Grosz and Zimmerman 1965; Theodor and Mandelcorn 1973). The auditory system may be affected, leading to deafness or auditory hallucinations, the latter being the most common form of hallucinations in conversion disorder (Aplin and Kane 1985).

The sense of touch can be affected, producing anesthesias, analgesias, or even tactile hallucinations. The distribution of symptoms follows an idiosyncratic pattern that does not reflect neuroanatomical sensory distribution. This gives rise to "glove" or "stocking" distribution patterns, which commonly affect either the upper or lower extremities. Hemianesthesias are also seen, with a clear sensory loss that stops in the midline and commonly involves an entire side of the body. A historically notorious but uncommon presentation in modern times is "devil's patches," which consists of idiosyncratic areas of sensory loss, usually around the genitals. In the days of witch hunts, these were considered a demonic sign and used as proof of the victims' pact with the devil. This symptom may be associated with traumatic events such as accidents or sexual abuse.

Sensory dysfunction may also consist of pain, which tends to be 1) localized to the abdominal cavity, 2) localized to the genital areas, or 3) have the pattern of a fatal illness. If pain is a symptom of conversion disorder, other symptoms must also be present. If the symptoms are limited to pain, pain disorder would be a more appropriate diagnosis (assuming the criteria for that disorder are met).

Seizures or Convulsive Phenomena (Pseudoseizures)

Conversion seizures or pseudoseizures (also referred to as nonconvulsive seizures or nonepileptic events) are characterized by 1) variable onset, which is usually gradual; 2) relatively prolonged duration (compared with epileptic seizures), often lasting minutes to hours; 3) greater frequency of occurrence than epileptic seizures; 4) a tendency to occur in the presence of others; and 5) a link with an acute environmental stressor (Ramani et al. 1980; Roy 1980; Theodore 1989) (Table 4–2).

Patients usually exhibit bizarre and unusual behavior, have no electroencephalogram (EEG) abnormalities, lack postictal confusion, and recall what occurred during the pseudoseizure (Desai et al. 1982; Ramani et al. 1980). Body movements are random, uncoordinated, purposeful, asynchronous, and appear to consist of consciously integrated motor activity. Often, the wild and dis-

Table 4–2.   Characteristics of psychogenic seizures or pseudoseizures

Behavior during seizure activity is wide in range and bizarre in character.

Electroencephalogram (EEG) recording is usually normal during and after seizure activity.

There is usually no relationship between seizure activity and anticonvulsant medication or blood levels.

Onset of seizure activity is usually gradual.

Duration of the seizure is usually prolonged.

A primary and/or secondary gain may be identified.

Postictal confusion is absent.

Seizures may be reproduced or triggered by suggestion or suggestive techniques.

Recollection of the events that took place during the seizure usually ranges from good to intact.

Seizures usually occur in older children or adults.

Tongue biting, urinary incontinence, and injuries during seizures are rare.

No abnormal neurological signs or reflexes are present during or immediately after the seizure.

Seizures rarely occur during sleep.

The frequency of pseudoseizures is usually much higher than epileptic seizures.

organized thrashing of the "convulsion" appears, to the observer, to be a theatrical caricature of a true seizure.

Given the psychogenic nature of the episodes, patients rarely experience physical injuries (such as tongue biting or head trauma), almost never experience incontinence, rarely show elevation in serum prolactin levels, and rarely benefit from anticonvulsive therapy. In fact, patients usually present with a history of resistance to conventional pharmacotherapy. Pseudoseizures are common in neurology settings, accounting for one-half of inpatient evaluations and one-fifth of outpatient epilepsy clinic visits (Riley and Berndt 1980).

Most psychogenic seizures can be grouped into one of two categories, depending on the form of epileptic activity that they resemble (Krumholz and Niedermeyer 1983; Ramchandani and Schindler 1993; Veith 1965). "Major pseudoseizures," which are seen in about two-thirds of cases, consist of seizure activity that mimics generalized tonic-clonic phenomena or myoclonic seizures. Symptoms of "minor pseudoseizures" include those resembling absence or partial complex seizures. Approximately one-third of patients present with a combination of major and minor seizure activity.

About one-half of patients referred by neurologists to psychiatrists to rule out pseudoseizures have nonepileptic seizures. However, between 37% and 42% of patients with "true epilepsy" have coexistent pseudoseizures (Krumholz and Niedermeyer 1983; Ramchandani and Schindler 1993).

Pseudoseizures are common in other psychiatric disorders, most often dissociative identity disorder (DID) (Putnam 1989; Putnam et al. 1986). This complicates matters, because one of the differential diagnoses of DID is temporal lobe epilepsy (Mesulam 1981; Schenk and Bear 1981).

Other Psychiatric Symptoms

In our clinical experience, a common symptom in patients with conversion disorder is a psychotic-like state (Spiegel and Fink 1979). It may be extremely difficult to differentiate this symptom from symptoms of a thought disorder during an acute episode. Conversion disorder should be suspected in patients with psychotic symptoms who are highly hypnotizable and who respond to hypnotic intervention during the psychotic state. Other features suggesting conversion psychosis include a lack of familial history of psychotic disorders; previous episodes of "psychosis" triggered by a stressor, with full remission after the stressor is removed and with little effect on the patient's subsequent functioning; and a history of somatization disorder or other conversion symptoms (Spiegel et al. 1982).

History

The diagnosis of DSM-IV-TR conversion disorder, known as conversion reaction in DSM-I and hysterical neurosis, conversion type, in DSM-II, entered psychiatric nosology in DSM-III. DSM-III clearly distinguishes somatization disorder, based on polysymptomatic complaints with symptoms related to various organs, from conversion disorder, based on monosymptomatic complaints with symptoms limited to motor or sensory functioning. Somatization involves anxiety about symptoms, whereas conversion emphasizes somatic dysfunction.

Even though the term "conversion disorder" is relatively new, conversion-like symptoms have been recognized for centuries (Table 4–3). Descriptions of the "wandering uterus" can be found in an ancient Egyptian medical text, *Kahun Papyrus* (Griffith 1897), written around 1900 B.C. Similarly, *Papyrus Ebers,* dating back to around 1600 B.C. and considered the greatest Egyptian medical document, has a chapter titled "Diseases of Women," which is devoted almost entirely to hysteria (Ebbell 1937). Both documents suggest that the origin of hysteria is associated with symptoms of the generative organs, specifically aberrations in the position of the womb. Hippocrates (circa 200 A.D.) believed that only women could have hysteria and that most female problems stemmed from the uterus as it "wandered throughout the body causing pain and disease." A dry uterus, for example, would "wander" about the body searching for moisture, causing great distress in the process. Hippocrates designed treatment strategies aimed at healing the uterus, including body bandaging intended to constrict movement of the uterus, potions and wine, and nasal and vaginal fumigations.

Galen (circa 200 A.D.) postulated that hysteria stemmed from the effects of "a vaporous sperm-like substance" secreted from the uterus. Hysterical symptoms occurred when the uterus was unable to appropriately eliminate this substance. Galen believed that sexual abstention in men could be manifested in a variety of physical symptoms, including shortness of breath, muscle paralysis or contractures, and seizures (Veith 1965). Galen also linked hysterical seizures to early sexual experiences (Goodwin et al. 1979).

In medieval times, the concept of "demonic possession" was used to explain major hysteria, a concept that served as the main model for conversion disorder throughout the 19th century. In

Table 4–3. Historical approaches to conversion disorder

Kahun Papyrus (circa 1900 B.C.)	Proposed that hysteria resulted from a "wandering uterus"
Papyrus Ebers (circa 1600 B.C.)	Proposed that hysteria resulted from a "wandering uterus"
Hippocrates (circa 200 A.D.)	Believed that only women could have hysteria
Galen (circa 200 A.D.)	Believed that sexual abstinence could trigger hysteria symptoms in men
Medieval times	Belief that demonic possession caused hysteria
Sydenham (1624–1680)	Described hysteria as a condition that mimics physical disease
Mesmer (1734–1815)	Proposed that imbalance in "magnetic fluid" caused hysteria symptoms
Raulin 1758	Introduced idea that men, not just women, can have hysteria
Briquet (1796–1881)	Postulated that hysteria resulted from stressful events that acted on the "affective part" of the brain
Reynolds 1869	Described hysteria as an illness that was based on an idea
Charcot (1825–1893)	Proposed that hysteria was caused by a degenerative neurological process
Janet (1859–1947)	Postulated that hysteria could be attributed to dissociation
Bernheim (1889/1964)	Postulated that hypnotizability and suggestibility were exhibited by all individuals
Breuer and Freud (1893–1895/1955)	Described hysteria as the result of an uncontrolled hypnotic-like state mediated by repression and as the result of repression of intrapsychic conflicts

fact, even today, some accounts of demonic possession have a conversion-like quality to their presentation. It is likely that throughout history, conversion phenomena have been mistaken for supernatural phenomena occurring in highly suggestible individuals.

Thomas Sydenham (1624–1680), who in the 17th century advanced the modern notion of hysteria as a psychological disorder, described hysteria as "a condition that could mimic all the physical diseases to which man is heir" (Sydenham 1666; see also Latham 1848). Raulin (1758), one of Sydenham's disciples, first introduced the idea that men (not only women, as originally believed) could also experience hysterical illnesses.

Franz Anton Mesmer (1734–1815), whose theory of "magnetic fluid" later became known as mesmerism (Goldsmith 1934; Walmsley 1967) and then hypnosis, suggested that nervous and mental disorders, including hysterical symptoms, could be produced when the ebb and flow of this fluid within a person was out of harmony with the universal rhythm.

In the early 19th century, Paul Briquet (1796–1881) published what is considered the "first general work of real value [in hysteria]," which "prepared the way for the contemporary studies" (Janet 1907). Briquet (1859) developed the modern concept of hysteria as a chronic polysymptomatic disorder and provided the first known systematic description of its characteristics. Briquet attributed the phenomena of hysteria to a "dysfunction of the nervous system" and postulated that the disorder was the result of stressful events that acted on the "affective part" of the brain of vulnerable individuals. Closely following Briquet's ideas are those of Reynolds (1869), who eloquently described clinical cases in which he attributed pain or loss of function to an "idea that the patient had about his or her body." It was Reynolds who first described "illness behavior dependent on an idea."

The famous French neurologist Jean Martin Charcot (1825–1893) had a different view of the symptoms of hysteria. Expanding on the theories of Briquet and Reynolds, Charcot (1890) suggested that hysteria occurred only in individuals "with a brain predisposed by heredity." Charcot proposed that "a traumatic event led to an idea that caused a functional or dynamic lesion in the brain" (Havens 1966; see also Chertok 1984). His thoughts on hysteria and conversion defined theories on the origins of hysteria for years. Charcot (1889) postulated that hysteria represented a special state of consciousness in which individuals actually experience their lack of functions or anesthesia as real. His followers and contemporaries, however, including Bernheim (1889/1964), Janet (1907), and Breuer and Freud (1893–1895/1955), refuted the organic basis of Charcot's ideas, attributing the symptoms of conversion to unconscious mechanisms rather than true neurological conditions.

At the beginning of the 20th century, Pierre Janet (1859–1947) continued to study hysteria and developed the basis for modern theories of conversion disorder. Janet expanded on Reynold's concept of an idea as an underlying mechanism leading to a pathological state, departing from the neurological theories of his teacher, Charcot. Janet postulated that the basis for conversion disorder could be dissociation, building a theory of the unconscious involving compartmentalization of memory. According to this dissociative model, information kept out of awareness is relatively untransformed and can be accessed directly using techniques such as hypnosis.

According to Janet, the major symptoms of hysteria are somnambulism, double personalities, convulsive attacks, contractures, paralyses, anesthesia, and hysterical stigmata, as well as disturbances of speech, vision, alimentation, and respiration. Janet (1920, 1925) promoted the concept that ideas and affects may be lost to consciousness, but somehow continue to exert sensory and motor effects via unconscious mechanisms. Janet held Charcot's views on the degenerative neural basis for hysteria. Later, Bernheim (1889/1964) challenged the ideas of Charcot and Janet by postulating that hypnotizability and suggestibility were exhibited by individuals without hysteria and therefore do not represent a disease process.

Sigmund Freud, who was exposed to Charcot's work and later influenced by Bernheim, worked with Josef Breuer and discovered that while in a trance, some patients with hysterical symptoms could recall past traumatic memories and emotional experiences that were related and probably causative of patients' symptoms. Freud and Breuer were the first to use the term "conversion" to refer to the substitution of a somatic symptom for a repressed idea (Jones 1953). They also described how the recollections of these repressed memories led to symptom relief (Freud 1958). Thus, Freud and Breuer began to use hypnotic age regression or hypnotic reenactment (the precursor of the cathartic method) to treat hysterical symptoms. This led to the development of their theory linking unconscious determinants to conscious symptoms. Freud and Breuer believed that "hypnoid-like" states constituted the building blocks of hysterical symptomatology, recognizing that hypnotic processes are normal and yet can be mobilized to resolve an unconscious conflict. This led to the theory of "conservation of psychic energy," which proposed that emotion that could not be expressed otherwise would be "converted" into physical symptoms. In other words, the affect associated with traumatic events, which was not expressed because of the moral or ethical meaning to the patient, could be repressed and converted into a somatic hysterical symptom that was symbolic, in some way, of the original emotional trauma. The purpose of therapy was to uncover the traumatic memories and associated affects (abreaction) so that emotional catharsis could occur, resulting in symptom resolution.

Freud later expanded on these principles, stating that the repressed affects and conflicts were often sexual in nature and usually involved real or fantasized seduction by the patient's father. Subsequent psychoanalytic theories on hysterical conversion became an extension of Freud's early theories of the Oedipal phase of psychosexual development. Even though the original Freudian concept of conversion primarily focused on conflicts over sexuality, themes of conflicts over aggressive impulses and dependency needs are also accepted in the current psychodynamic understanding of conversion phenomena.

Guze developed Briquet's descriptive diagnosis of medically unexplained somatic symptoms, which he named Briquet's syndrome (Guze and Perley 1963). Guze (1970) formulated a list of diagnostic criteria for the disorder that was modified by and introduced into DSM-III as somatization disorder. The current DSM-IV-TR diagnosis of somatization disorder preserves much of Guze's description of the disorder.

Models of Symptom Generation

There have been numerous theories about the etiology of conversion disorder. Current thinking is strongly influenced by dissociative and psychodynamic models that emphasize repression.

As previously noted, Janet (1920) introduced the dissociative model. According to this model, information is kept out of awareness in a relatively untransformed manner but continues to exert sensory and motor effects via unconscious mechanisms, which cause hysterical and other dissociative symptoms. Freud's previously described principle of conversion and repression model of hysteria suggested that psychological conflicts too difficult to process consciously are "converted" or transformed into physical symptoms. Kardiner and Spiegel (1947) described the traumatic etiology of conversion symptoms and posttraumatic disorders associated with combat experience. They conceptualized such conversion symptoms as a nonverbal language of action, or the expression of conflict over fear and loyalty to comrades, resulting in apparent physical dysfunction that provided an honorable exit from an intolerable situation (Spiegel 1974). They also demonstrated the usefulness of hypnosis in diagnosing and treating both posttraumatic stress disorder and conversion symptoms.

Barr and Abernethy (1977) posited a behavioral approach to understanding conversion symptoms, suggesting that "conversion is an adaptation to a frustrating life experience." Similarly, Celani (1976) described conversion symptoms as "the result of cultural, social, and interpersonal influences," and the way the patient has "learned to communicate helplessness, thereby facilitating an environment in which attention and support are gained and aggressive impulses avoided." Celani suggested that secondary gains are common in conversion disorder by stating that "the patient's symptoms may be reinforced by the reactions of caretakers and families [secondary gains] perpetuating symptoms and symptom formation during times of stress and conflict." Ford and Folks (1985) described conversion symptoms as a form of "primitive communication via pantomime when direct verbal communication is blocked." These more modern theories are not entirely different from the original theories proposed by Bernheim, Janet, Breuer, and Freud, but they utilize more behavioral or mechanistic language.

Hurwitz (1989) suggested that conversion symptoms depend on a patients' "conscious participation and are produced by a conscious enactment of ideas of illness." His views radically departed from the classic psychoanalytic theories, which suggest that unconscious mechanisms involve a split in consciousness, or dissociation, because of the individual's inability to express affect, which is transformed into a physical symptom (Breuer and Freud 1893–1895/1955). Hurwitz used drug disinhibition or a "go–no go paradigm" to support his theory. Although his sample was very small, Hurwitz was able to temporarily help his patients recover normal functioning. He believed that recovery of function depended on distraction in which "the schema of the affected body part was no longer in the patient's field of conscious attention." Thus, Hurwitz believed that patients consciously generated their symptoms—modeling them after their own previous illnesses or similar processes in other family members—to signal distress because they were unable to express themselves in linguistic or psychological terms, or because they believed that physical symptoms were more acceptable than psychological distress.

Regardless of the underlying pathogenic mechanism, the diagnosis of conversion disorder may be complicated by some patients' tendency to model their symptoms after their own physical illnesses. Watson and Buranen (1979) called this "a paralogical extension of physical disease." That is, patients may mimic symptoms they experienced in the past (paralogical extension) or may unconsciously replay the symptoms experienced by a significant person (object) (symptom identification) (Lazare 1978; Lewis and Berman 1965). Or, as postulated in the "learned behavior" theory, symptoms learned during childhood are later used in adult life to cope with particular situations (Barr and Abernethy 1977).

Ludwig (1972) and Whitlock (1967) proposed "centrifugal inhibition of afferent stimuli" as a mechanism for conversion symptoms. Flor-Henry et al. (1981), using data from neuropsychological testing batteries, suggested that symptoms could be explained as "a concrete representation of ideas blocked from verbal expression." Furthermore, Flor-Henry and colleagues suggested an impairment of both dominant and nondominant cerebral hemispheres, with greater deficit in the dominant one. We have suggested (Maldonado 1996) that a process associated with "unconscious hyperattention" or "unconscious monitoring" may explain certain types of conversion disorder.

Finally, some have criticized the validity of the diagnosis of conversion disorder. Even Charcot stated that "malingering is to be found in every phase of hysteria" (Merskey 1979). Thus, critics of the diagnosis have suggested that the symptoms of hysteria (conversion) are factitiously created because they are an acceptable way to enact the sick role, thus avoiding certain responsibilities and manipulating the behavior of others (Celani 1976; Halleck 1967; Rabkin 1964). According to DSM-IV-TR, such symptoms do not meet criteria for conversion disorder.

Functions Served by Conversion Symptoms

The symptoms of conversion disorder appear to serve a number of unconscious purposes. These include permitting oneself to express a forbidden wish or impulse in a masked form, imposing punishment on oneself via a disabling symptom for a forbidden wish or wrongdoing, removing oneself from an overwhelming life-threatening situation (primary gain), and assuming the sick role to allow gratification of dependency needs (secondary gain).

The last function listed needs to be differentiated from the primary goal of being in the sick role, which is characteristic of factitious disorder, and the secondary gains of malingering. In conversion disorder, the symptoms are secondary to the repression or dissociation of memories and/or affect. Instead of feeling the pain associated with certain affects, the pseudoneurological symptoms maintain the dissociation of affect from the memories. The mechanism by which the symptoms are produced is not consciously available to the person who experiences them. Thus, patients see themselves as victims of their symptoms. The secondary gains are by-products of the conversion symptoms. The main goals of symptom production are the symbolic resolution of unconscious conflicts and an attempt to keep the conflicting memories out of consciousness. This leads to prevention or reduction of anxiety (primary gain).

In contrast, in factitious disorder, symptoms are consciously produced, with the goal of placing oneself in the sick role (Maldonado, in press). Although external incentives (e.g., disability) may be present, as in the case of conversion disorder, they are not the primary motivating factor. In malingering, symptoms are consciously produced with the primary intent of obtaining some tangible external objective (secondary gain), such as avoiding work, military draft, or criminal prosecution, or obtaining drugs or financial compensation.

Finally, as discussed previously, a function served by conversion symptoms is communication (Barr and Abernathy 1977; Celani 1976). There usually appears to be a hidden message in the language of conversion symptoms, which communicates the patient's frustration, anger, hatred, sorrow, and guilt.

> Mr. L, who was driving his mother in his car, approached an intersection and could not see oncoming traffic on the right. As he entered the intersection, Mr. L noticed a large truck approaching the passenger side of his car. He tried to avoid the truck; however, the truck hit the car, killing his mother. Mr. L underwent a comprehensive panel of laboratory and diagnostic tests, including computed tomography (CT) of his head and neck. He had superficial lacerations on his forehead and scalp, a broken left arm, and a chest contusion. Results of a neurological examination were within normal limits. The only symptom that could not be explained was his blindness. Results of magnetic resonance imaging (MRI) of his head were normal, with no defects observed in the occipital area that would explain his blindness. A hypnotic approach was suggested to deal with Mr. L's anxiety and assist with the diagnostic process. Using a dissociative technique called the "television technique," in which he visualized events as if were observing them on an imaginary television screen, Mr. L was able to reexamine the events of the accident. He then realized his responsibility for the accident. Further exploration during subsequent sessions allowed Mr. L to express his guilt and remorse and how he had arrived at his own punishment: "It was my fault. I didn't see the truck. If I can't see, I'll never kill again." Under hypnosis, Mr. L allowed himself to "see" again. The scene of the accident was reconstructed, but instead of "everything going blank" he was allowed to stay conscious and "see" his mother and the emergency personnel's attempts to rescue her. He was given suggestions to allow himself to recover his vision whenever he was ready. Mr. L was able to see again after three sessions.

Associated Features

Clinical features associated with conversion disorder include a history of conversion episodes or Briquet's syndrome (somatization disorder). In some cases, symptom identification may be present; that is, the conversion symptoms appear to be modeled after an important figure in the patient's life (Lazare 1978; Lewis and Berman 1965). In some cases, exploration of the family history reveals a family member with an illness after which the patient's symptoms are modeled (e.g., paralysis as identification with a grandparent who uses a wheelchair). Alternatively, the symptoms may follow a pattern of an injury or physical deficit previously experienced by the patient (paralogical extension), such as convulsions modeled after febrile seizures.

As previously noted, primary gain may be identified, which may be associated with sexual conflicts, feelings of guilt, or aggressive impulses for which the patient feels he or she should be punished. Similarly, some secondary gains resulting from being sick may be evident. A study by Raskin et al. (1966) found an 86% incidence of secondary gains in patients with conversion disorder, compared with 22% in those presenting with organic disease. However, many patients, regardless of their diagnosis, may experience some degree of secondary gain; thus, this is not a useful diagnostic feature. In addition, secondary gain may be difficult to reliably identify.

The early literature on hysteria and conversion emphasizes the presence of "la belle indifference." This refers to an inappropriate cavalier attitude or lack of concern about the nature or implications of a serious symptom or condition. Conversely, patients may present with exaggerated or histrionic symptoms. However, the so-called "hysterical personality" is rarely seen in association with conversion disorder. A longitudinal study by Lempert and Schmidt (1990) found that the prevalence of hysterical personality features in patients with conversion disorder was as low as 8%.

Epidemiology, Demographic Features, and Disease Course

Although the incidence and prevalence of conversion disorder is not clear, various authors report rates ranging from 11/100,000 to 500/100,000 in the general population (American Psychiatric Association 2000; Ford and Folks 1985; Toone 1990). The annual incidence of conversion disorder in patients seen by general psychiatrists has been reported to be as low as 0.01%–0.02% (Barsky 1989). On the other hand, studies have indicated that the lifetime prevalence may be as high as 5%–14% among general hospital inpatients receiving psychiatric consultation (Barsky 1989; Folks et al. 1984; McKegney 1967; Stefansson et al. 1976a; Stoudemire 1988). The rates of some specific forms of conversion have been reported to be even higher. For example, the incidence of psychogenic seizures have ranged from 8%–24% (Krumholz and Niedermeyer 1983; Ramchandani and Schindler 1993).

In specialized settings, the rate of conversion disorder has been found to be high. Of patients admitted to general hospital neurology wards for evaluation of seizures, 44% received a diagnosis of psychogenic seizures (Sumner et al. 1952). In that same study, 55% of patients admitted for evaluation of pseudoseizures received this diagnosis. In general, psychogenic seizures have been described as occurring in 8%–24% of neurology patients with intractable seizures (Desai et al. 1982; Krumholz and Niedermeyer 1983; Lempert and Schmidt 1990; Peterson et al. 1950; Ramani et al. 1980; Ramchandani and Schindler 1993; Sumner et al. 1952; Trimble 1986).

Conversion disorder has been reported to be 2–5 times more common in women than in men (Barsky 1989; Ljundberg 1957; Stefansson et al. 1976a). Some reports suggest that the rate may be 10 times higher in women (Bowman 1993; Raskin et al. 1966). In a longitudinal outpatient study of pseudoseizures, 71% of patients were women (Krumholz and Niedermeyer 1983). In a study of conversion seizures, 64% of patients were women (Lempert and Schmidt 1990). In the sample of patients with pseudoseizure studied by Bowman (1993), 92% were women. Conversion symptoms in men are often associated with a history of an industrial, occupational, or military accident (Allodi 1974; Carden and Schamel 1966; Kardiner and Spiegel 1947; Rabkin 1964).

The onset of conversion disorder can occur at any age but most commonly occurs during adolescence and early adulthood. Onset before age 10 is rare (Maloney 1980). Occurrence of the disorder after age 80 has been reported (Weddington 1979). Age at first consultation among pseudoseizure patients in a neurology clinic ranged from 15 to 78 years, with a mean of 38 years (Lempert and Schmidt 1990). The mean age at onset has been reported to be later for men (around age 25) than for women (around age 17). Some data suggest that there may be a pattern of familial aggregation (Ljundberg 1957). Limited data also suggest that the risk of conversion disorder is higher in monozygotic twin pairs than dizygotic twin pairs (Inouye 1972). Anecdotal evidence suggests a tendency for the disorder to occur more frequently in the youngest child in the family. Some studies have reported a higher incidence of conversion disorder among low socioeconomic groups, rural populations, and individuals with little education or limited knowledge of medical or psychological concepts (Folks et al. 1984; Guze and Perley 1963; Stefansson et al. 1976b; Weinstein et al. 1969).

The onset of conversion disorder is usually acute, with variable progression of symptoms. Often the onset occurs at or after the occurrence of significant stressors. Symptom duration is often relatively brief, with remission usually occurring within 2 weeks if the stressor is removed or addressed. Carter (1949) reported that 90 (90%) of 100 patients were fully recovered by the time of hospital discharge. According to Ford and Folks (1985), approximately 25 (50%) of 50 conversion patients experienced complete symptom resolution by the end of their hospital stay. Carter (1949) followed 100 patients for 4–6 years and found that 73 (73%) were doing well by the end of the study. Similarly, Hafeiz (1980) found that after 1-year follow-up, only 12 (20%) of 61 recovered patients had experienced a relapse of conversion symptoms. On the other hand, the condition sometimes has a remitting and relapsing course. In approximately 20%–25% of cases, symptoms recur within a year after the initial episode. In a study by Kent et al. (1995), 66 (67%) of 98 patients diagnosed with conversion disorder met diagnostic criteria at 4-year follow-up. The most likely explanations for the differences in these rates include the diversity of the patient populations, differences in diagnostic criteria used, differences in symptom presentation (e.g., paralysis versus pseudoseizures), and the sophistication of the medical technology and other diagnostic techniques available at the time.

The prognosis is good for patients of above-average intelligence who have an acute presentation that clearly follows a stressor and who receive early, aggressive psychiatric intervention. Patients with paralysis or aphonia or whose symptoms are associated with the senses (e.g., blindness, deafness) also have a good prognosis. On the other hand, patients who experience a subacute presentation, diagnostic and therapeutic delay, tremors, and pseudoseizures are associated with poor prognosis (Ford and Folks 1985).

Comorbidity

Conversion disorder commonly occurs in association with other psychiatric and medical disorders (Bowman 1993). Psychiatric disorders commonly seen in patients with conversion disorder are major depression, somatization disorder (Briquet's syndrome), anxiety disorders, alcohol abuse, dissociative disorders, depersonalization disorder, and personality disorders. The most common lifetime psychiatric diagnosis in patients with acute conversion symptoms is major depression (about 85%) (Roy 1980; see also Zeigler et al. 1960). In a study of 26 patients with pseudoseizure, Bowman (1993) found a high rate of current psychiatric disorders and history of trauma, with a history of sexual abuse or rape in 77% and a history of physical abuse in 70%. Eighty-five percent had depressive disorders, 85% had dissociative disorders, 33% had posttraumatic stress disorder, and 11% had panic attacks. The most common personality disorders in women with conversion disorder are histrionic and dependent personality disorders, according to DSM-III-R. Among men with conversion disorder, antisocial personality disorder is the most common Axis II diagnosis, as reported in DSM-IV and by Allodi (1974) and Robins et al. (1952).

A number of neurological conditions are associated with conversion disorder. One study found that approximately 70% of patients diagnosed with conversion disorder had evidence of a preceding or coexisting neurological disorder (Barsky 1989). In another study, neurological disorders were identified in 44% of patients with conversion symptoms (Krumholz and Niedermeyer 1983). However, Folks et al. (1984) found that the incidence of true medical or neurological problems in their sample was low (about 20%). The most common neurological or medical finding is a history of head trauma. In one study, 25% of men and 11% of women had a history of head injury (Ljundberg 1957). Bowman (1993) reported that 66% of patients reported a history of head injuries, 55% of which were severe enough to cause loss of consciousness. EEG abnormalities have been reported in 38% of patients with psychogenic seizure; these abnormalities were attributed to organic neurological disorders or anticonvulsant drug toxicity (Krumholz and Niedermeyer 1983). Other neurological diagnoses associated with conversion symptoms include the following:

- Multiple sclerosis
- Central nervous system tumors
- Intelligence quotient (IQ) less than 80, which occurred in 17% of patients studied by Krumholz and Niedermeyer (1983)
- True seizure disorders (Ramchandani and Schindler 1993), which occurred in 37%–42% of patients studied by Krumholz and Niedermeyer (1983)

It is especially important for psychiatrists who consult on cases of suspected conversion disorder to keep these figures in mind and avoid premature closure regarding a diagnosis of functional versus organic disease. Looking for neurologic comorbidity will decrease the risk of misdiagnosis. A misdiagnosis of conversion disorder may prevent a patient from obtaining an adequate medical work-up or treatment.

Differential Diagnosis

It is imperative that patients suspected of having conversion disorder receive a thorough neurological and medical evaluation. As previously discussed, neurologic conditions may coexist with conversion disorder. In their follow-up study, Gatfield and Guze (1962) found that the conversion symptoms of 21% of patients diagnosed with conversion disorder were actually attributable to neurologic disease. Slater and Glithero (1965) reported that 30% of patients originally diagnosed with conversion disorder were found to have organic illness that apparently accounted for their original presentation. Other studies found that less than 30% of cases of conversion disorder were incorrectly attributed to a medical cause (Carter 1949; Dickes 1974; Folks et al. 1984; Hafeiz 1980). It is important to keep in mind that patients diagnosed with conversion disorder may have an undiagnosed or unrecognized medical illness and that up to 70% will eventually develop a disease that might in some way explain the pathology initially presented.

The incidence of misdiagnosis may be declining. Watson and Buranen (1979) found after a 10-year follow-up period that 25% of diagnoses of conversion disorder were in fact false-positive diagnoses. In a more recent 4-year follow-up study, Kent et al. (1995) found that only 13% of patients were initially misdiagnosed. Even though the rate of misdiagnosis has declined, these studies confirm that medical illness continues to be the cause of the original presenting complaint in a substantial number of patients initially diagnosed with conversion disorder. For this reason, it is imperative that patients thought to have conversion disorder receive a thorough neurological and medical evaluation. Conversion disorder should not be considered a diagnosis of exclusion. Rather, it is a well-defined entity that mimics neurological processes. On the other hand, the presence of a neurological condition does not preclude the diagnosis of conversion disorder. In fact, as previously noted, some studies indicate that conversion symptoms may occur in patients who have a true organic disorder. Possible organic disorders to consider include mostly occult or difficult-to-diagnose neurological disorders, which may mimic or present with primarily neurological symptoms. These include systemic lupus erythematous, myasthenia gravis, multiple sclerosis, Parkinson's disease, a true seizure disorder, and the effects of various medications, drugs of abuse, and alcohol on the central nervous system.

At the same time, it is important that medical and neurologic disorders not be overdiagnosed. Studies show that there is an average of 6–8 years' delay before conversion disorder is diagnosed

(Bowman 1993), usually because of previous misdiagnosis of and treatment for medical, neurological, or other psychiatric conditions. Some diagnostic tests may actually cause iatrogenic damage, which in turn may validate the patient's perceived deficits. Similarly, some medications (e.g., benzodiazepines, anticonvulsants, neuroleptics) may promote depersonalization, dissociative states, mental slowing, or a "hangover" effect, which patients may misunderstand and which may further promote their feeling of lack of control.

Psychiatric diagnoses that should be considered and ruled out before diagnosing conversion disorder include pain disorder and sexual dysfunction (both of which are diagnoses of exclusion according to DSM-IV-TR Criterion F). Other psychiatric diagnoses that may better explain the symptoms are psychotic disorders (in the case of hallucinations or psychotic presentation, including nonculturally sanctioned psychotic-like presentations), anxiety disorders (in the case of shortness of breath or difficulty swallowing), dissociative disorders (because they share symptoms such as dissociation and neurological dysfunction or changes), and the other somatoform disorders (e.g., somatization disorder and hypochondriasis). Finally, as previously discussed, the possibility of factitious disorder or malingering must be considered.

Treatment

The treatment of patients with conversion disorder is best carried out in collaboration with an internist, primary care physician, or neurologist. In most cases, neither medical nor psychiatric treatment alone suffices. A joint approach is often best, which includes adequate medical intervention directed at diagnosing the cause of the patient's symptoms. After ruling out medical problems or managing any that are present, psychiatric consultation is indicated. The first step in treating conversion disorder involves reassuring the patient that the symptoms are not the result of a medical or neurological condition, but are secondary to an underlying psychological conflict. However, it is wise to present this information to patients and their families in a manner that does not imply that the patients have been faking their symptoms or that their symptoms do not have a physical component. Rather, an approach that conveys that there are physical and psychological aspects of the illness that can best be addressed by a rehabilitation approach invites the patient to engage in treatment without feeling humiliated (Spiegel and Chase 1980). Clinical experience suggests that a brief psychotherapeutic intervention directed at placing the symptoms, their meaning, and their implications in context may be helpful. Addressing the stressors that may have led to onset, including any identified trauma, is paramount to an effective intervention. On the other hand, there is seldom a need to "go on a fishing expedition." Allowing the patient to make any connections that might be present between current stressors and earlier conflicts, and recognizing the need to address them by working on developing more adaptive defenses, is usually adequate. The adjunctive use of relaxation techniques, with or without hypnosis training, may be beneficial.

If symptoms do not improve or resolve with this conservative approach, more intensive intervention may be needed. This may include a number of techniques used alone or jointly, including a pharmacologically facilitated interview (i.e., narcoanalysis), behavioral therapies, and hypnosis. As already discussed, the faster the resolution of the presenting symptoms, the better the prognosis appears to be.

Narcoanalysis has been described as an effective technique in the management of acute conversion symptoms (Ford 1995; Grinker and Spiegel 1945; Horsley 1943; Hurwitz 1988, 1989; Kolb 1985; Marcos and Trujillo 1978; Perry and Jacobs 1982; Tureen and Stein 1949). Many authors have suggested that narcoanalysis has limited utility in cases of chronic conversion symptoms (Cloninger 1993; Ford 1995; Hurwitz 1988; Kolb 1985). It should be used only when more conservative approaches, such as placement in a protective environment and reassurance, have failed. The use of barbiturates (amytal or pentobarbital) has declined in favor of the short-acting benzodiazepines (lorazepam), given their greater margin of safety. There are few risks when narcoanalysis is used to relieve the patient's distress, is limited to discussion of any acute stressors leading to the conversion, and is used to enhance a sense of control. A potential problem with this or any other method of memory enhancement is the risk of "going on a fishing expedition," trying to find early psychological traumas that may account for present symptoms. This approach increases the risk of memory contamination. Because of potential legal ramifications of the use of any method of memory enhancement, adequate training and supervision is recommended. Maldonado et al. (1997) discussed methods of memory enhancement, including narcoanalysis and hypnosis, and the risks of using them.

The use of a number of behavioral techniques is similar to their use in other psychiatric disorders and has been discussed elsewhere (Ford 1983, 1995; Wickramasekera 1997, 1999). Behavioral techniques combine a protective environment, reassurance that a full medical work-up has concluded that no permanent damage has been found and that full recovery is expected, and relaxation techniques (e.g., biofeedback, relaxation training). As is the case with hypnosis, suggestive techniques are usually incorporated as part of the behavioral treatment and include reassurance that the symptoms will improve rapidly and in fact are already beginning to improve.

Hypnosis is a form of heightened concentration, an alert state of focused awareness, with concomitant physical relaxation (Spiegel and Spiegel 1987), which may be useful in treating conversion disorder. A patient with hypnotic potential can be easily trained to achieve this state of concentration (trance state). After an appropriate patient is trained in self-hypnotic techniques, he or she can be helped to develop the skills needed to manipulate some of his or her own bodily sensations and functions.

Charcot (1890) reported an association between conversion disorder and high hypnotic capacity He first described how hypnosis not only could alleviate conversion symptoms but also could reproduce them. More recently, Bliss (1984) reported that patients with conversion disorder are very hypnotizable, and other studies have corroborated that such patients are more highly hypnotizable than the population at large. For example, studies have indicated that only 20%–30% of the general population is highly hypnotizable, compared with nearly 70% of patients with psychogenic seizures (Peterson et al. 1950). We hypothesize that patients with conversion disorder may be using their capacity to dissociate to displace the uncomfortable feelings or affects into a chosen part of the body, which then becomes dysfunctional. Thus, hypnosis may be useful in both the diagnosis and treatment of conversion symptoms (Barry et al. 2000; Bowman 1993; Bush et al. 1992; Maldonado 1996; Maldonado and Jasiukaitis, submitted for publication).

Hypnosis should be used as an adjunct to, rather than in lieu of, medical treatment. Hypnosis is not used to remove conversion symptoms but to allow patients to control the effects of emotional stress and mind states on their bodily functions. Therefore, it is not appropriate to use hypnosis to cure a patient with conversion disorder. In fact, an attempt to forcefully remove a symptom usually results in worsening of the original symptom or the formation of new ones (uncontrolled symptom substitution). Patients often develop symptom substitution, usually characterized by symptoms that are more severe than the original ones, when their defenses are threatened. A more effective approach is to train patients to use self-hypnotic techniques and allow them to improve at a pace that is comfortable for them, while the clinician provides suggestions for improved control and mastery and explores the unconscious psychological reasons behind the presence of symptoms, including the possibility of secondary gain. The therapist adopts the role of a coach guiding the patient through the process rather than doing things for the patient. The patient is helped through the process of understanding the nature, meaning, and usefulness of the symptoms and is given the necessary tools to cope with the deficits and to "give up" symptoms when ready.

The use of hypnosis to treat conversion disorder involves several phases. The first phase involves exploring the meaning of the symptoms. It is important to never eliminate a symptom without understanding its purpose and replacing it with a more adaptive defense. The second phase involves symptom alteration (i.e., taking the patient's mind away from the presenting symptoms while allowing him or her to find more appropriate ways to cope with anxiety). This may be accomplished by symptom substitution, in which a given symptom is exchanged for another, which is less impairing or pathological until the patient is ready to give up the original symptom (e.g., replacing the perception of intense cancer pain with a numbing, tingling sensation in the same area), or symptom extinction, in which the patient agrees to give up the symptom after working through the problem in psychotherapy. The third phase involves maximizing the patient's level of functioning. Hypnosis may be used to increase the patient's motivation, enhance his or her sense of mastery, and strengthen his or her defenses.

Conclusion

Conversion disorder dramatically illustrates the complex relationships among mind, brain, and body. Symptoms often appear after the occurrence of stressors, reflecting the impact of such events on the brain and mind. Conversion symptoms may also co-occur with neurological or physical illness, or as a way to identify with illness in a loved one. Inability to understand or express emotion may trigger conversion symptoms, and certain kinds of social contact may reinforce them. There is reason for therapeutic optimism, because psychological and social input may also ameliorate or eliminate symptoms. Psychotherapies of various types are effective in altering and eliminating symptoms while helping the patient work through stress-related problems. A variety of therapeutic approaches that teach patients how to enhance control over somatic processes by altering, ameliorating, or eliminating conversion symptoms can reduce symptoms while addressing related problems and stressors.

References

Allodi FA: Accident neurosis: whatever happened to male hysteria? Canadian Psychiatric Association Journal 19:291–296, 1974

American Psychiatric Association: Diagnostic and Statistical Manual: Mental Disorders. Washington, DC, American Psychiatric Association, 1952

American Psychiatric Association: Diagnostic and Statistical Manual of Mental Disorders, 2nd Edition. Washington, DC, American Psychiatric Association, 1968

American Psychiatric Association: Diagnostic and Statistical Manual of Mental Disorders, 3rd Edition. Washington, DC, American Psychiatric Association, 1980

American Psychiatric Association: Diagnostic and Statistical Manual of Mental Disorders, 4th Edition. Washington, DC, American Psychiatric Association, 1994

American Psychiatric Association: Diagnostic and Statistical Manual of Mental Disorders, 4th Edition, Text Revision. Washington, DC, American Psychiatric Association, 2000

Aplin DY, Kane JM: Variables affecting pure tone and speech audiometry in experimentally simulated hearing loss. Br J Audiol 19:219–228, 1985

Barr R, Abernethy V: Conversion reaction. Differential diagnoses in the light of biofeedback research. J Nerv Ment Dis 164:287–292, 1977

Barry JJ, Atzman O, Morrell MJ: Discriminating between epileptic and nonepileptic events: the utility of hypnotic seizure induction. Epilepsia 41:81–84, 2000

Barsky AJ: Somatoform disorders, in Comprehensive Textbook of Psychiatry/V, 5th Edition, Vol 1. Edited by Kaplan HI, Sadock BJ. Baltimore, MD, Williams & Wilkins, 1989, pp 1009–1027

Bernheim H: Hypnosis and Suggestion in Psychotherapy: A Treatise on the Nature of Hypnotism (1889). Translated by Herter CA. New Hyde Park, NY, University Books, 1964

Bliss EL: Hysteria and hypnosis. J Nerv Ment Dis 172:203–206, 1984

Bowman ES: Etiology and clinical course of pseudoseizures. Relationship to trauma, depression, and dissociation. Psychosomatics 34:333–342, 1993

Breuer J, Freud S: Studies on hysteria (1893–1895), in The Standard Edition of the Complete Psychological Works of Sigmund Freud, Vol 2. Translated and edited by Strachey J. London, Hogarth Press, 1955, pp 1–311

Briquet P: Traité clinique et thérapeutique à l'hystérie. Paris, J-B Balliere and Fils, 1859

Bush E, Barry JJ, Spiegel D, et al: The successful treatment of pseudoseizures with hypnosis (letter). Epilepsia 33:135, 1992

Carden NL, Schamel DJ: Observations of conversion reactions seen in troops involved in the Viet Nam conflict. Am J Psychiatry 123:21–31, 1966

Carter AB: The prognosis of certain hysterical symptoms. British Medical Journal 1:1076–1079, 1949

Celani D: An interpersonal approach to hysteria. Am J Psychiatry 133:1414–1418, 1976

Charcot JM: Clinical Lectures on the Diseases of the Nervous System, Vol 3. Translated by George Sigerson. London, New Sydenham Society, 1889

Charcot JM: Oeuvres Completes de JM Charcot, Tome IX. Paris, Lecrosnier et Babe, 1890

Chertok L: On the centenary of Charcot: hysteria, suggestibility and hypnosis. Br J Med Psychol 57:111–120, 1984

Cloninger CR: Somatoform and dissociative disorders, in Medical Basis of Psychiatry, 2nd Edition. Edited by Winokur G, Clayton PJ. Philadelphia, WB Saunders, 1993, pp 169–192

Deary IJ, Wilson JA, Mitchell L, et al: Covert psychiatric disturbance in patients with globus pharynges. Br J Med Psychol 62:381–389, 1989

Desai BT, Porter RJ, Penry JK: A study of 42 attacks in six patients, with intensive monitoring. Arch Neurol 39:202–209, 1982

Dickes RA: Brief therapy of conversion reactions. Am J Psychiatry 131:584–586, 1974

Ebbell B (trans): The Papyrus Ebers, the Greatest Egyptian Medical Document. Copenhagen, Levin and Munksgaard, 1937

Fallik A, Sigal M: Hysteria—the choice of symptom site: a review of 40 cases of conversion hysteria. Psychother Psychosom 19:310–318, 1971

Farley J, Woodruff RA, Guze SB: The prevalence of hysteria and conversion symptoms. Br J Psychiatry 114:1121–1125, 1968

Flor-Henry P, Frown-Augh D, Tepper M, et al: A neuropsychological study of the stable syndrome of hysteria. Biol Psychiatry 16:601–626, 1981

Folks DG, Ford CV, Regan WM: Conversion symptoms in a general hospital. Psychosomatics 25:285–289, 1984

Ford CV: The Somatizing Disorders: Illness as a Way of Life. New York, Elsevier, 1983, pp 49–72

Ford CV: Conversion disorder and somatoform disorder not otherwise specified, in Treatments of Psychiatric Disorders, 2nd Edition, Vol 2. Edited by Gabbard GO. Washington, DC, American Psychiatric Association, 1995, pp 1735–1753

Ford CV, Folks DG: Conversion disorders: an overview. Psychosomatics 26:371–383, 1985

Freud S: Remembering, repeating, and working-through (further recommendations on the technique of psycho-analysis II) (1914), in The Standard Edition of the Complete Psychological Works of Sigmund Freud, Vol 2. Translated and edited by Strachey J. London, Hogarth Press, 1958, pp 145–156

Gatfield PD, Guze SG: Prognosis and differential diagnosis of conversion reactions (a follow-up study). Diseases of the Nervous System 23:623–631, 1962

Goldsmith M: Franz Anton Mesmer: The History of an Idea. 1934.

Goodwin J, Simms M, Bergman R: Hysterical seizures: a sequel to incest. Am J Orthopsychiatry 49:698–703, 1979

Griffith FI: The Petri Papyri, in Hieratic Papyri from Kahun and Gurob, Vol I: Literary, Medical and Mathematical Papyri from Kahun. London, Bernard Quaritch, 1897, pp 5–11

Grinker RB, Spiegel JP: Men Under Stress. Philadelphia, Blakiston, 1945

Grosz HJ, Zimmerman J: Experimental analysis of hysterical blindness. Arch Gen Psychiatry 13:255–260, 1965

Guze SB: The role of follow-up studies: their contribution to diagnostic classification as applied to hysteria. Seminars in Psychiatry 2:392–402, 1970

Guze SB, Perley MJ: Observations on the natural history of hysteria. Am J Psychiatry 119:960–965, 1963

Hafeiz HB: Hysterical conversion: a prognostic study. Br J Psychiatry 136:548–551, 1980

Halleck SL: Hysterical personality traits. Arch Gen Psychiatry 16:750–757, 1967

Havens L: Charcot and hysteria. J Nerv Ment Dis 141:505–516, 1966

Horsley JS: Narcoanalysis. New York, Oxford Medical Publications, 1943

Hurwitz TA: Narcosuggestion in chronic conversion symptoms using combined intravenous amobarbital and methylphenidate. Can J Psychiatry 33:147–152, 1988

Hurwitz TA: Ideogenic neurological deficits: conscious mechanisms in conversion symptoms. Neuropsychiatry Neuropsychol Behav Neurol 1:301–308, 1989

Inouye E: Genetic aspects of neurosis. International Journal of Mental Health 1:176–189, 1972

Janet P: The Major Symptoms of Hysteria. New York, Macmillan, 1907, 1920

Janet P: Psychological Healing: A Historical and Clinical Study. New York, Macmillan, 1925

Jones E: The Life and Work of Sigmund Freud. New York, Basic Books, 1953

Kardiner A, Spiegel H: War Stress and Neurotic Illness. New York, Paul Hoeber, 1947

Kent DA, Tomasson K, Coryell W: Course and outcome of conversion and somatization disorders. A four-year follow-up. Psychosomatics 36:138–144, 1995

Kolb LC: The place of narcosynthesis in the treatment of chronic and delayed stress reactions of war, in The Trauma of War. Edited by Sonnenberg SM, Blank AS, Talbott JA. Washington, DC, American Psychiatric Press, 1985

Krumholz A, Niedermeyer E: Psychogenic seizures: a clinical study with follow-up data. Neurology 33:498–502, 1983

Latham RG (trans): The Works of Thomas Sydenham, M.D. London, 1848

Lazare A: Hysteria, in MGH Handbook of General Psychiatry. Edited by Hackett TP, Cassem NH. St Louis, Mosby, 1978, pp 117–140

Lazare A: Current concepts in psychiatry. Conversion symptoms. N Engl J Med 305:745–748, 1981

Leigh BC, Riley WT: The psychiatric management of globus syndrome. Gen Hosp Psychiatry 9:214–219, 1988

Lempert T, Schmidt D: Natural history and outcome of psychogenic seizures: a clinical study in 50 patients. J Neurol 237:35–38, 1990

Lewis WC, Berman M: Studies of conversion hysteria: operational study of diagnosis. Arch Gen Psychiatry 13:275–282, 1965

Ljundberg L: Hysteria: clinical, prognostic and genetic study. Acta Psychiatr Scand Suppl 32:1–162, 1957

Ludwig AM: Hysteria: a neurobiologic theory. Arch Gen Psychiatry 27:771–777, 1972

Maldonado JR: Physiological correlates of conversion disorders. Paper presented at the annual meeting of the American Psychiatric Association, New York, May 1996

Maldonado JR: Factitious disorders: when patients deceive themselves and their doctors. American Journal of Forensic Psychiatry (in press)

Maldonado JR, Jasiukaitis P: Selective attention in conversion disorders (submitted for publication)

Maldonado JR, Butler LD, Spiegel D: Treatment of dissociative disorders, in A Guide to Treatments That Work. Edited by Nathan PE, Gorman JM. London, Oxford University Press, 1997, pp 423–446

Maloney MJ: Diagnosing hysterical conversion disorders in children. J Pediatr 97:1016–1020, 1980

Marcos LR, Trujillo M: The sodium amytal interview as a therapeutic modality. Current Psychiatric Therapies 18:129–136, 1978

McKegney FP: The incidence and characteristics of patients with conversion reactions: a general hospital consultation service sample. Am J Psychiatry 124:542–545, 1967

Merskey H: The Analysis of Hysteria. London, Bailliere Tindall, 1979

Mesulam M-M: Dissociative states with abnormal temporal lobe EEG. Arch Neurol 38:176–181, 1981

Miller E: Detecting hysterical sensory symptoms: an elaboration of the forced choice technique. Br J Clin Psychol 25:231–232, 1986

Perry JC, Jacobs D: Overview: clinical applications of the amytal interview in psychiatric emergency settings. Am J Psychiatry 139:552–559, 1982

Peterson DB, Sumner JW, Jones GA: Role of hypnosis in differentiation of epileptic from convulsive-like seizures. Am J Psychiatry 107:428–433, 1950

Pilowsky I: Abnormal illness behavior. Br J Med Psychol 42:347–351, 1969

Puhakka HJ, Kirveskari P: Globus hystericus: globus syndrome? J Laryngol Otol 102:231–234, 1988

Putnam FW: Diagnosis and Treatment of Multiple Personality Disorder. New York, Guilford, 1989

Putnam FW, Guroff JJ, Silberman EK, et al: The clinical phenomenology of multiple personality disorder: review of 100 cases. J Clin Psychiatry 47:285–293, 1986

Rabkin R: Conversion hysteria as a social maladaptation. Psychiatry 27:349–363, 1964

Ramani SV, Quesney LF, Olson D, et al: Diagnosis of hysterical seizures in epileptic patients. Am J Psychiatry 137:705–709, 1980

Ramchandani D, Schindler B: Evaluation of pseudoseizures. A psychiatric perspective. Psychosomatics 34:70–79, 1993

Raskin M, Talbott JA, Meyerson AT: Diagnosis of conversion reactions: predictive value of psychiatric criteria. JAMA 197:530–534, 1966

Raulin J: Traite des affections vaporeuses d'un sexe avec l'exposition de leurs symptomes, de leurs differentes causes et la methode de les guerir. Paris, 1758

Reismann JL, Singh B: Conversion reactions simulating Guillain-Barre paralysis following suspension of the swine flu vaccination program in the U.S.A. Aust N Z J Psychiatry 12:127–132, 1978

Reynolds JR: Paralysis and other disorders of motion and sensation dependent on idea. BMJ 2:483–485, 1869

Riley TL, Berndt T: The role of the EEG technologist in delineating pseudoseizures. American Journal of EEG Technology 20:89–96, 1980

Robins E, Purtell JJ, Cohen ME: "Hysteria" in men. N Engl J Med 246:677–685, 1952

Roy A: Hysteria. J Psychosom Res 24:53–56, 1980

Schenk L, Bear D: Multiple personality and related dissociative phenomena in patients with temporal lobe epilepsy. Am J Psychiatry 138:1311–1316, 1981

Slater ET, Glithero E: A follow up-of patients diagnosed as suffering from "hysteria." J Psychosom Res 9:9–13, 1965

Spiegel H: The grade 5 syndrome: the highly hypnotizable person. Int J Clin Exp Hypn 22:303–319, 1974

Spiegel D, Chase RA: The treatment of contractures of the hand using self-hypnosis. J Hand Surg [Am] 5:428–432, 1980

Spiegel H, Spiegel D: Trance and Treatment: Clinical Uses of Hypnosis. Washington, DC, American Psychiatric Press, 1987

Spiegel D, Fink R: Hysterical psychosis and hypnotizability. Am J Psychiatry 136:777–781, 1979

Spiegel D, Detrick D, Frischholz E: Hypnotizability and psychopathology. Am J Psychiatry 139: 431–437, 1982

Stefansson JG, Messina JS, Meyerowitz S: Hysterical neurosis, conversion type: clinical and epidemiological considerations. Acta Psychiatr Scand 53:119–138, 1976a

Stefansson JG, Markidis M, Christodoulou G: Observations on the evolution of hysterical symptomatology. Br J Psychiatry 128:269–275, 1976b

Stoudemire AG: Somatoform disorders, factitious disorders, and malingering, in The American Psychiatric Press Textbook of Psychiatry. Edited by Talbott JA, Hales RE, Yudofsky SC. Washington, DC, American Psychiatric Press, 1988, pp 533–556

Sumner JW, Cameron RR, Peterson DB: Hypnosis in differentiation of epileptic from convulsive-like seizures. Neurology 27:395–402, 1952

Sydenham T: Methodus curandi febres, propriss observationibus superstructa, in Transactions of the Royal Society. London, 1666

Theodor LH, Mandelcorn MS: Hysterical blindness: a case report and study using a modern psychophysical technique. J Abnorm Psychol 82:552–553, 1973

Theodore WH: Pseudoseizures: differential diagnosis. J Neuropsychiatry Clin Neurosci 1:67–69, 1989

Toone BK: Disorders of hysterical conversion, in Physical Symptoms and Psychological Illness. Edited by Bass C. London, Blackwell Scientific, 1990, pp 207–234

Trimble MR: Pseudoseizures. Neurol Clin 3:531–548, 1986

Tureen LL, Stein M: The base section psychiatric hospital. Bulletin of the US Army Medical Department 9(suppl):105–137, 1949

Veith I: Hysteria: The History of a Disease. Chicago, IL, University of Chicago Press, 1965

Walmsley DM: Anton Mesmer. London, Ebenezer Baylis and Sons, 1967

Watson CG, Buranen C: The frequency and identification of false positive conversion reactions. J Nerv Ment Dis 167:243–247, 1979

Weddington WW Jr: Conversion reaction in an 82-year-old man. J Nerv Ment Dis 167:368–369, 1979

Weinstein EA, Eck RA, Lyerly OG: Conversion hysteria in Appalachia. Psychiatry 32:334–341, 1969

Whitlock F: The aetiology of hysteria. Acta Psychiatr Scand 43:144–162, 1967

Wickramasekera I: Secrets kept from the mind, but not the body, and behavior: somatoform disorders and primary care medicine. Biofeedback Fall:20–22, 1997

Wickramasekera I: How does biofeedback reduce clinical symptoms and do memories and beliefs have biological consequences? Toward a model of mind-body healing. Appl Psychophysiol Biofeedback 24:91–105, 1999

Wilson JA, Deary IJ, Maran GD: Is globus hystericus? Br J Psychiatry 153:335–339, 1988

Wilson JA, Deary IJ, Maran GD: The persistence of symptoms in patients with globus pharyngitis. Clin Otolaryngol 16:202–205, 1991

World Health Organization: The ICD-10 Classification of Mental and Behavioural Disorders: Clinical Descriptions and Diagnostic Guidelines. Geneva, World Health Organization, 1992

Ziegler FJ, Imboden JB, Meyer E: Contemporary conversion reactions: a clinical study. Am J Psychiatry 116:901–910, 1960

Chapter 5

Factitious Disorder

Marc D. Feldman, M.D.
James C. Hamilton, Ph.D.
Holly N. Deemer, M.A.

Nearly every physician and mental health professional has heard of factitious disorder (FD), though many know the disorder only by the more evocative name of the most extreme subtype, Munchausen syndrome. FD is diagnosed in persons who intentionally exaggerate or induce signs and symptoms of physical or mental illness or who pretend to be physically or mentally ill when they are not. By definition, these pretenses are not motivated by financial gain or other obvious benefit (DSM-IV-TR; American Psychiatric Association 2000). FD has been described in more than 2,000 published case reports, and accounts of the more dramatic cases sometimes appear in the popular media. Health professionals and the lay public alike are captivated by the bizarre accounts of persons who poison, infect, or injure themselves in some way to gain admission to hospitals and even to be subjected to painful and potentially dangerous medical and surgical procedures. Equally captivating are the accounts of people who feign depression, dissociative disorder, or dementia to assume the role of psychiatric patient.

In this chapter, we will summarize what is known about the basic clinical features of FD. We will also present some of the diagnostic issues raised by current approaches to FD and discuss differential diagnosis, comorbidity, costs, and prevalence. We will conclude by reviewing current theories of the etiology of FD and clinical observations about strategies for managing and treating FD patients. Throughout, we will try to avoid adding to the medical literature yet another review of this disorder. Instead, we will offer a critique of the FD literature that questions the way FD is conceptualized in current nosological systems, and we will try to delineate the methodological problems that must be solved in order to arrive at a scientifically sound understanding of FD. We will argue that there is little to be gained, and much to be lost, by the use of the current practice of viewing the somatoform disorders, factitious disorder, and malingering as discreet and distinct clinical entities. We will argue for the working hypothesis that all cases of unexplained medical complaints (UMCs) fall along a wide continuum of what we call "factitious illness behavior," which we define as sick role behavior that is not motivated by the desire to maintain or restore physical or mental health. According to this view, there are a number of biopsychosocial factors that contribute to FD and, across all cases, these factors operate in varying combinations and to varying degrees. Perhaps this dimensional view of FD will shift attention away from the current emphasis on categorizing FD and toward the goal of understanding the underlying psychopathology of FD and related disorders.

Epidemiology and Etiology

Before beginning our overview of FD, we will describe briefly the state of the empirical literature on the epidemiology and etiology of FD. We provide this information so that the reader can put into proper context the clinical description of FD that we present.

We performed a MEDLINE search for all indexed articles published between 1966 and May 2000 that contained the terms "factitious" or "Munchausen." The search yielded 2,155 citations. Additional searches were performed to determine the proportion of these articles that presented empirical evidence related to the clinical epidemiology or etiology of FD. The results of these searches are presented in Table 5–1. More than half the articles do not contain an abstract; therefore, we assumed that they are letters, editorials, or comments and excluded them. More than two-thirds of the remaining articles presented case reports. Of the remaining 201 citations, most presented general observations about FD cases or general information about diagnosing and managing

Table 5–1. MEDLINE articles containing the term "factitious" or "Munchausen" published between 1966 and May 2000

	Number of articles	Articles remaining
Articles containing the terms "factitious" or "Munchausen"	2,155	2,155
Articles without abstracts	1,480	675
Case reports	474	201
Summaries, reviews, and tutorials	175	26

FD. Only 26 articles could be defined as systematic attempts to collect data about, and draw inferences from, multiple cases (defined as 3 or more). Seven of the 26 articles reported the prevalence of FD in a large sample of medical patients (e.g., the percentage of patients with fever of unknown origin who had FD) (Knockaert et al. 1992; Rumans and Vosti 1978; Sarwari and Mackowiak 1997). Thirteen articles described the medical, demographic, or psychiatric characteristics of a sample of FD patients. Although we found 3 case-controlled studies that compared the prevalence of FD in patients and control subjects, we could find only 1 case-controlled study that compared the characteristics of FD patients and control subjects (Craven et al. 1994). All but 6 of the studies were retrospective chart reviews. Only 2 studies described FD cases in terms of psychological assessments not ordinarily included in the routine documentation of medical cases. To our knowledge, there has never been any federal funding of FD research.

In sum, there is very little empirical evidence related to the epidemiology of FD and almost none related to the etiology of FD. Four books on patient deception (Feldman and Eisendrath 1996; Feldman and Ford 1994; Ford 1996; Pankratz 1998) draw inferences based on consolidations of published reports and clinical experience, but evidence is still heavily anecdotal. Thus, despite the fact that the medical community has recognized factitious ailments for more than a century (Gavin 1843) and that FD has received considerable attention since then, the scientific study of FD has not meaningfully progressed beyond the use of the case study method.

There are two complementary reasons for the lack of empirical research on FD. First, it is very difficult to study easily identified cases of FD. Second, it is very difficult to identify easily studied cases. Patients who we are certain have met the criteria for FD typically have simulated or induced an illness to gain admission to a hospital. In these cases, it is sometimes possible to uncover definitive physical evidence (e.g., from laboratory tests) that the patient's illness is factitious. However, patients who have engaged in this degree of fraudulent sick role behavior may face civil liability or even criminal prosecution for defrauding hospitals or their health insurance companies or providers (Feldman 1995; Risse et al. 1992). For this reason and others, patients are seldom willing to submit to psychiatric assessments or psychological study, and they often flee the hospital or sign out against medical advice. On the other hand, patients who engage in less blatant forms of FD, such as exaggerating or simply lying about discomfort or disability, are much more amenable to participating in research studies. However, in these cases it is nearly impossible to determine definitively that their illness behavior is factitious. What may appear to be gratuitous sick role behavior may be motivated by fear (as in hypochondriasis) or may reflect an as-yet-undiscovered physical disease or mental disorder.

Although rich in clinical information, published case reports represent an unsystematic sample probably biased toward more extreme examples of FD. In addition, the information in these reports is not standardized in a way that would permit aggregation. Beyond the inclusion of simple demographic data and a description of the patient's deception, there is little consistency from one case report to the next. Medical specialists write most reports for the narrow purpose of alerting their peers to a particular method of feigning a particular disease. Only a minority of the reports addresses the psychosocial aspects of the case.

Despite its limitations, for now we must work with the descriptive information about FD that has been derived from clinical experience with FD cases. However, it is important to keep in mind that most of the material we present has yet to be confirmed through large-scale epidemiological studies of FD. In the last section of this chapter, we will suggest several strategies for promoting this empirical research.

Diagnosis

DSM-IV-TR recognizes four subtypes of factitious disorder (Tables 5–2 and 5–3): FD with predominantly physical signs and symptoms (300.19); FD with predominantly psychological signs and symptoms (300.16); FD with combined physical and psychological signs and symptoms (300.19); and FD not otherwise specified (300.19). For each of these disorders, the primary diagnostic criterion is the presence of signs or symptoms of physical and/or psychological illness that are feigned or produced. Each of these diagnoses depends on the ability of the clinician to affirm that the ailments are intentionally falsified or produced, and to confirm the absence of any external (e.g., material) incentives for adopting the sick role. If external incentives are present, the behavior is regarded as malingering (Cunnien 1988; Eisendrath 1996b; Plewes and Fagan 1994).

Table 5–2. DSM-IV-TR diagnostic criteria for factitious disorder

---

A. Intentional production or feigning of physical or psychological signs or symptoms.
B. The motivation for the behavior is to assume the sick role.
C. External incentives for the behavior (such as economic gain, avoiding legal responsibility, or improving physical well-being, as in Malingering) are absent.

Code based on type:

> **300.16   With Predominantly Psychological Signs and Symptoms:**   if psychological signs and symptoms predominate in the clinical presentation
>
> **300.19   With Predominantly Physical Signs and Symptoms:**   if physical signs and symptoms predominate in the clinical presentation
>
> **300.19   With Combined Psychological and Physical Signs and Symptoms:**   if both psychological and physical signs and symptoms are present but neither predominates in the clinical presentation

---

Table 5–3. DSM-IV-TR description of factitious disorder not otherwise specified

This category includes disorders with factitious symptoms that do not meet the criteria for factitious disorder. An example is factitious disorder by proxy: the intentional production or feigning of physical or psychological signs or symptoms in another person who is under the individual's care for the purpose of indirectly assuming the sick role.

Source. Reprinted with permission from American Psychiatric Association: *Diagnostic and Statistical Manual of Mental Disorders*, 4th Edition, Text Revision. Washington, DC, American Psychiatric Association, 2000, p. 517. Copyright 2000, American Psychiatric Association.

ICD-10 diagnostic criteria (World Health Organization 1992) (Table 5–4) are similar to DSM-IV-TR criteria, with several important exceptions. First, DSM-IV-TR criteria include no items related to the duration or frequency of the factitious illness behavior; therefore, by those criteria, a person can be diagnosed with FD on the basis of a single incident of factitious illness behavior. Second, ICD-10 Criterion C may discourage clinicians from diagnosing FD in patients who are exaggerating an otherwise authentic illness. Third, the DSM-IV-TR narrative description of FD explicitly differentiates self-mutilation, in which the patient does not lie about the origins of his or her injury, from FD, in which the patient does attempt to deceive the clinician. ICD-10 does not make this distinction. Finally, ICD-10 includes the stipulation that the motivation of "gaining more medical care" is an external incentive and thus would indicate malingering, not FD. In most cases, this incentive would be viewed as internal under DSM-IV-TR. ICD-10 criteria are weakened by the implication that one can reliably distinguish the pursuit of the gratifications of the sick role from the pursuit of more medical care.

Clinical Description

Subtypes and a Continuum of Severity

In addition to the subtypes of FD in DSM-IV-TR, there are distinctions that can be made among FD cases. Perhaps the most frequent

Table 5–4. ICD-10 diagnostic criteria for intentional production or feigning of symptoms of disabilities, either physical or psychological [factitious disorder]

A. The individual exhibits a persistent pattern of intentional production or feigning of symptoms and/or self-infliction of wounds in order to produce symptoms.
B. No evidence can be found for an external motivation, such as financial compensation, escape from danger or more medical care.
C. Most commonly used exclusion clause. There is no confirmed physical or mental disorder that could explain the symptoms.

Source. Reprinted with permission from *World Health Organization: International Statistical Classification of Diseases and Related Health Problems,* 10th Revision. Geneva, World Health Organization, 1992. Copyright 1992, World Health Organization.

source of confusion in the nomenclature of FD is the misuse of the term "Munchausen syndrome." Although many clinicians use Munchausen syndrome (Asher 1951) as a synonym for FD, the term is more accurately used to describe a severe and chronic subtype of FD (American Psychiatric Association 2000; Faguet 1980; Fink and Jensen 1989; Ludwigs et al. 1994). Patients with Munchausen syndrome are singularly dedicated to playing the sick role. These patients manipulate their bodies to simulate or induce physical illness or injury in an attempt to gain admission to a hospital for medical care. The maladies may be so esoteric that most physicians have little familiarity with them. When patients' deceptions are uncovered, the patients play out their role at other hospitals in the same city or another, thus repeating the pattern (peregrination). Munchausen patients also classically present with pseudologia fantastica (Hardie and Reed 1988; King and Ford 1988; Newmark et al. 1999), telling grand lies about their educational or military credentials, their past exploits, their social or political connections, and so forth. The use of aliases sometimes occurs (Meagher and Collins 1997). Thus, Munchausen syndrome is defined by the triad of 1) a severe and chronic course of FD, 2) peregrination, and 3) pseudologia fantastica. It characterizes 10% of FD patients (Reich and Gottfried 1983).

Eisendrath (1996a) reported that approximately two-thirds of patients with Munchausen syndrome are male, but that females outnumber males by 3:1 in the non-Munchausen forms of factitious physical disorders.

In contrast to the description of the prototypical Munchausen patient, it is believed that the majority of patients with FD lead relatively routine lives, although personality disorders (especially DSM-IV-TR Cluster B) and interpersonal problems are common among these patients. The typical FD patient is female, is often employed in a health-related field, and has a relatively unremarkable social and family life (Bock and Overkamp 1986; Eisendrath 1996b; Ford 1983; Reich and Gottfried 1983). Although FD patients may present with a chronic pattern of sick role behavior, for many patients the factitious behavior occurs episodically, presumably in response to negative life events. Medically dangerous methods of inducing or simulating illness are less common among typical FD patients than among patients with Munchausen syndrome (Eisendrath 1996b).

Methods of Simulating or Inducing Factitious Illnesses

It would be useful if there were a short and exclusive list of illnesses that FD patients feign. Unfortunately, one fact that has emerged from published cases of FD is that almost any illness or injury can be falsified or induced. Table 5–5 presents a partial list of factitious physical signs, symptoms, and illnesses that were documented in 199 case reports of FD published between 1996 and 1999. An exhaustive list of medical disorders that have been feigned or produced by FD patients would approximate the length of an index of a pathology textbook. The array of reported psychological manifestations is summarized in Table 5–6.

Although practically any disorder can be enacted or created in FD, there is a subset of medical conditions that appears repeatedly in the case literature. The most common clinical problems feigned or produced both in factitious physical disorders as a whole and in Munchausen syndrome are infection, impaired wound healing, hypoglycemia, anemia, bleeding, rashes, neurologic symptoms such as seizures or dizziness, vomiting, diarrhea,

Table 5–5. Factitious physical signs, symptoms, and illnesses documented in 199 case reports of factitious disorder published between 1996 and 1999

Acromegaly	Gastrointestinal bleeding	Periodontal injury
Acute respiratory distress	Gingival injury	Persistent discharge from arthroscopic portals
Bartter's syndrome	Hemoptysis	Pheochromocytoma
Blepharokeratoconjunctivitis (chronic)	HIV disease	Pulmonary talcosis
Breast cancer	Hypertensive crisis	Purpura
Burns	Hypocalcemia	Quadriplegia
Cervicofacial subcutaneous emphysema	Infectious diseases (various)	Rash
Cheilitis	Intra-alveolar pulmonary siderophages	Rectorrhagia
Connective tissue diseases	Lymphedema	Reflex sympathetic dystrophy
Cushing's syndrome	Malaria	Renal colic
Deafblindness	Malignancy	Seizures
Dermatoses	Maxillofacial injuries	Sickle cell acute painful episodes
Diabetes mellitus	Methemoglobinemia	Thrombocytopenia
Diphenhydramine poisoning	Mutilation of the hand	Urinary calculi
Diplopia	Necrotizing fasciitis	Vaginal bleeding
Epidermolysis bullosa simplex	Orbital emphysema	

Table 5–6. Presentations in factitious disorder with predominantly psychological signs and symptoms

Amnesia	Hallucinations or delusions
Bereavement	Hypersomnia
Bipolar disorder	Pain disorder
Cognitive impairment	Paraphilias
Depression	Posttraumatic stress disorder
Dissociative identity disorder	Substance-related disorder
Eating disorder	Transsexualism

Source. Adapted with permission from Parker PE: "Factitious Psychological Disorders," in *The Spectrum of Factitious Disorders.* Edited by Feldman MD, Eisendrath SJ. Washington, DC, American Psychiatric Press, 1996, p. 40. Copyright 1996, American Psychiatric Press.

pain or fever of undetermined origin, and symptoms of autoimmune or connective tissue disease (American Psychiatric Association 2000; Feldman and Ford 1994). It is likely that the FD patient's choice of disease reflects a careful balance between the desire to effectively deceive medical staff and to command their avid attention and concern. Subjective complaints of pain or weakness are virtually impossible to disprove, but they are unlikely to cause prolonged or intensive concern among medical staff. On the other hand, self-administered injections of anticoagulant medications will produce alarming signs and symptoms that the medical staff cannot ignore, but the patient runs the risk that the deception will be discovered as a result of the avid scrutiny. The most common factitious psychological disorders appear to be bereavement, cognitive impairment, depression, posttraumatic stress disorder, pain disorder, and dissociative identity disorder.

The foregoing analysis might suggest the FD patients would not feign disorders for which there are definitive tests, but the case literature suggests that this is not so. Even disorders for which there exist definitive medical tests have been convincingly feigned. For example, several dozen case reports describe patients who successfully feigned not only HIV-positive status but also AIDS (Craven et al. 1994; Joseph-Di Caprio and Remafedi

1997; Zuger and O'Dowd 1992). In these cases, the patients looked and played the part of an AIDS patient so convincingly that their physicians did not feel the need to corroborate the patients' reports of well-established HIV seropositivity.

The methods used to simulate or produce illnesses or injuries are as diverse as the medical conditions themselves. These methods can be grouped into five categories (Folks et al. 2000):

1. Exaggerations of pain, discomfort, and disability
2. Lies about the presence of various signs and symptoms of illness or injury, or dramatic enactments of these signs and symptoms (e.g., fake seizures)
3. Attempts to tamper with test instruments or with blood, stool, or urine samples to produce positive test results
4. Manipulations of one's physical condition to produce positive test results (e.g., introducing blood into the bladder) or other signs and symptoms of illness (e.g., using a tourniquet to cause limb edema)
5. Manipulations that cause actual physical harm (e.g., infecting oneself through self-injection with bacteria)

From case reports, it is clear that patients with FD are likely to employ several of these methods. For example, a patient pretending to have meningitis may complain of headaches and a stiff neck and ingest a pyrogenic substance to produce fever. It is also possible that, in individual cases, the course of a factitious illness reflects the use of progressively more dramatic and convincing methods as the medical staff begins to doubt the truth of the patient's self-reports. There are no reliable data on the frequency with which FD patients employ each of these methods, however.

Associated Features

DSM-IV-TR points to possible predisposing factors to FD. These include the presence of other mental disorders or general medical conditions during childhood or adolescence that led to extensive medical treatment and hospitalization; family disruption or emotional and/or physical abuse in childhood; a grudge against the medical profession; employment in a medically related position; and the presence of a severe personality disorder, particularly borderline personality disorder.

To assist in diagnosis, a number of experts in clinical practice and in medicolegal consultation have gone beyond DSM-IV-TR criteria to advocate the pragmatic use of indicators, or common characteristics, that have been observed repeatedly in confirmed cases of FD with predominantly physical signs and symptoms (Eisendrath et al. 1996). Such lists have proved helpful when applied to reviews of all available information (especially written records) in a specific case, though they have not been empirically evaluated for their reliability and validity. One such list is provided in Table 5–7. There are additional indicators that are relevant to factitious psychological disorders:

- The patient's symptoms and signs are inconsistent with the known features of the mental disorder, sometimes being displayed as a patent caricature.
- New symptoms that arise are remarkably similar to those exhibited by other patients on the ward or in the clinic.
- If alleged physical, sexual, and/or emotional trauma is involved, no witnesses corroborate the patient's story.
- If deaths of loved ones are claimed (as in factitious bereavement), they are purported to have been especially dramatic or gruesome and are unverifiable.

Evidence exists for isolated cases of feigned psychosis, but such patients often develop authentic psychotic disorders when followed longitudinally (Suresh and Srinivasan 1990). Indeed, feigning a psychosis may be a defense against the emergence of a genuine psychosis (Cunnien 1988).

Prevalence

There are no published prevalence rates of FD in the population at large, and reliable data on the prevalence of FD in medical populations are scarce. Eckhardt-Henn (1999) estimated the prevalence of FD in general medicine to be between 0.5% and 2.0% of

Table 5–7. Indicators of factitious disorder on chart review

Signs and symptoms are not controllable. There is continual escalation, improvement is reliably followed by relapse, or new complaints are elaborated to keep caregivers engaged.

The magnitude of symptoms consistently exceeds objective pathology and/or there is proved exaggeration of symptoms by patient.

Some findings are determined to have been self-induced or at least worsened through self-manipulation.

There is a remarkable number of tests, consultations, and treatment efforts to little or no avail.

The patient is unusually willing to consent to medical/surgical procedures.

The patient disputes test results.

The patient predicts deteriorations, or there are exacerbations shortly before discharge.

The patient has sought treatment at numerous facilities.

The patient emerges as an inconsistent, selective, or misleading informant and/or he or she is resistant to allowing the treatment team access to outside information sources.

There is a history of medical intervention for secondary problems, which leads observers to state that the patient must be remarkably unlucky or accident-prone, or implies a significant psychogenic component.

Factitious disorder is explicitly considered by at least one health care professional.

The patient is noncompliant with diagnostic/treatment recommendations and/or is disruptive in the unit or the clinic.

The patient focuses on his or her self-perceived "victimization" by the medical and other systems.

There is evidence from laboratory or other tests that disputes information provided by the patient.

The patient prefers medical/surgical intervention to noninvasive treatment modalities.

The patient engages in gratuitous, self-aggrandizing lying.

While seeking medical/surgical intervention, the patient opposes psychiatric assessment.

There is evidence for motivations consistent with those known to have been important among confirmed factitious disorder patients.

Source. Adapted with permission from Eisendrath SJ, Rand DC, Feldman MD: "Factitious Disorders and Litigation," in *The Spectrum of Factitious Disorders.* Edited by Feldman MD, Eisendrath SJ. Washington, DC, American Psychiatric Press , 1996, p. 75. Copyright 1996, American Psychiatric Press.

all cases. Sutherland and Rodin (1990) reported that 0.8% of medical patients referred for psychiatric consultation had symptoms that met the criteria for FD. Kapfhammer et al. (1998b) reported a prevalence of 0.6% in a similar population. Although FD has been documented in nearly every medical specialty, FD may be particularly prevalent among certain patient groups. For example, Gault et al. (1988) found that 2.7% of kidney stones submitted for chemical analysis were not organic in origin, suggesting that patients had tried to pass off geologic stones as physiologic ones. Sabot (1999) arrived at a notably similar percentage. Ballas (1996) reported a prevalence of FD of 0.9% in a population of adolescents with sickle cell disease. As would be expected, the prevalence is particularly high among patients whose problems are inscrutable or intractable. In studies of patients with fever of unknown origin, prevalence estimates of FD have ranged from 2.2% to 9.3% (Aduan et al. 1979; Rumans and Vosti 1978). In a study comparing patients with brittle diabetes to a control group of patients with stable diabetes, "deliberate interference with therapy to induce diabetic instability was proven or admitted" in 40% of patients with poorly controlled diabetes and in 2% of patients with well-controlled diabetes (Gill 1992, p. 260). It is unclear how many of these patients had symptoms that would officially qualify for the diagnosis of FD; some may have been malingering. Fink (1992b) found that 20% of patients with a history of multiple UMCs had symptoms that met the diagnostic criteria for FD.

Table 5–8 presents reported prevalence rates of FD in various settings. Many of the studies were limited by diagnostic imprecision (e.g., whether an episode of illness was factitious or malingered, and whether—in cases involving children—the parent or patient engaged in the deceptions). Experts do concur that factitious physical disorders are most commonly observed in clinical practice, that the combined subtype is less common, and that the psychological variant is least common (American Psychiatric Association 2000).

Other investigators who have examined the prevalence of UMCs without regard to psychiatric diagnosis report much higher prevalence statistics (Bridges and Goldberg 1985; Kroenke and Mangelsdorff 1989). Even by the most conservative estimates,

Table 5–8. Prevalence of factitious disorder in various settings

Study	Setting	Size of study population	Illness	Number of cases	Prevalence of cases
Friedl and Draijer 2000	Consecutive psychiatric inpatients in the Netherlands over 1 year	122	Dissociative identity disorder	2	2%
Bogazzi et al. 1999	Endocrinology service at an Italian university hospital over 24 years	NA	Factitious thyrotoxicosis (surreptitious ingestion of thyroid hormone)	25	NA
Papadopoulos and Bell 1999	Neurosurgery inpatients at a London hospital over 8 years	18,893	Neurosurgical emergency	6	0.032%
Chua and Friedenberg 1998	Tertiary referral center in rural Wisconsin	11	Superwarfarin poisoning	2	18.2%
Kapfhammer et al. 1998a	German university hospital over 4 years	169	Pseudoneurologic signs	9	5.3%
Kapfhammer et al. 1998b	German university hospital over 18 years	15,000	Miscellaneous ailments	93	0.62%
Reich and Hanno 1997	Two Philadelphia-area hospitals	2,000	Renal colic	12	0.6%
Ballas 1996	Center for hematologic research in Philadelphia	NA	Sickle cell painful episodes	NA	0.9%
Bauer and Boegner 1996	Neurology service at a Berlin university hospital over 1 year	1,538	Neurologic syndromes	5	0.3%
Churchill et al. 1994	Specialty HIV unit in central London over 5 years	706	HIV infection	12	1.7%
Freyberger et al. 1994	Psychiatric consultation service at a general hospital in Germany over 10 years	NA	Miscellaneous ailments, especially wound healing disorders, hypoglycemia, anemia, and infection	70	NA
Knockaert et al. 1992	General medical service at a Belgian university hospital during the 1980s	199	Fever of unknown origin	7	3.5%

Table 5–8. Prevalence of factitious disorder in various settings *(continued)*

Study	Setting	Size of study population	Illness	Number of cases	Prevalence of cases
Fishbain et al. 1991	Pain and rehabilitation center in Florida	2,860	Chronic pain	4	0.14%
Sutherland and Rodin 1990	Psychiatric consultation service at a large teaching hospital in Toronto over 3 years	1,288	Miscellaneous ailments, mostly self-induced infection and trauma	10	0.8%
Bhugra 1988	Psychiatric hospital in England during 1 year (patients < age 65)	775	Psychiatric illness	4	0.5%
Gault et al. 1988	General hospital in Newfoundland	72[a]	Kidney stones	~ 9	~ 2.7% of stones were factitious
Dickinson and Evans 1987	Cardiac care unit of an inner-city London teaching hospital over 10 years	NA	Cardiac complaints	36	NA
Mohammed et al. 1985	Australian casualty department "black books" of "problem patients"	713	Miscellaneous ailments	21	2.9%
Reich and Gottfried 1983	Inpatients at a teaching hospital over 10 years	NA	Miscellaneous ailments	41	NA
Pope et al. 1982	U.S. research ward for psychotic disorders	219	Psychotic symptoms	9	4.1%
Aduan et al. 1979	National Institute of Allergy and Infectious Diseases	343	Fever of unknown origin	32	9.3%
Rumans and Vosti 1978	Stanford University Medical Center over 10 years	506	Fever of unknown origin	11	2.2%
Bunim et al. 1958	Adult and child patients at National Institutes of Health	200	Fever of unknown origin	13	6.5%

Note. NA = information not available.
[a]3,300 kidney stone specimens submitted by patients.

20%–30% of all medical visits are for medical complaints that have no objective physical basis. Although it is unclear how these cases of UMCs relate to FD, it is likely that some represent subclinical forms of factitious illness behavior. Support for this supposition is provided by Sansone et al. (1997), who reported that 7% of the primary care patients they studied admitted that they intentionally engaged in behavior that induced or prolonged an illness. It is unlikely that FD would be diagnosed in any of these cases, but it is highly likely that a large proportion of these patients engaged in some degree of factitious illness behavior.

Costs

The financial costs associated with FD are considerable. Case reports in which patients accumulate more than $100,000 in unnecessary medical costs are not uncommon (Donovan 1987; Feldman 1994; Powell and Boast 1993). Further costs can be attributed to the high health care utilization of persons with UMCs in whom the basic processes responsible for FD may play a role. In a comprehensive study of health care utilization in Denmark, Fink (1992a, 1992b) found that 56 patients with persistent somatization disorder accounted for 3% of the nonpsychiatric admissions for the entire population. Labott et al. (1995) estimated that patients with somatization disorder in a health maintenance organization (HMO) generated medical expenses that were 13 times higher than average. McCahill (1995) found that patients with somatization disorder generated hospital costs that were 6 times greater and ambulatory costs that were 14 times greater than those of control subjects. Ford (1992) estimated that the costs to society may be $20 billion annually. It is likely that a portion of these costs is attributable to mild to moderate forms of undiagnosed FD.

In addition to the financial costs of FD and related disorders, there are significant human costs. First, patients with FD, who repeatedly manipulate their physical condition to mimic or induce serious illness, face increased morbidity and mortality risks. FD also leads to iatrogenic risks associated with multiple unnecessary diagnostic and treatment procedures. These risks may be compounded by the failure of these patients to provide physicians with accurate information about their medical histories. Psychological costs are also exacted from doctors and nurses who experience frustration, anger, and demoralization when they learn that they have been duped by patients who have abused the health professionals' trust and caring (Feldman and Smith 1996). Finally, the existence of FD probably results in compromised care for patients who are genuinely ill, but whose illness presentations are atypical (Feldman and Ford 1994). Patients with systemic lupus, multiple sclerosis, and other idiopathic, variable, or unexpected illnesses may encounter health professionals who insinuate that their symptoms are psychogenic even though physical examination and evaluation has been notably incomplete (Rabins 1983).

Limitations of Current Approaches

All of the aforementioned costs of FD stem from the fact that practitioners do not have enough empirically based guidance to make accurate and timely diagnoses. Early identification and early intervention depend on the availability of valid, affirmative diagnostic criteria. However, for both FD and related disorders, there are no primary affirmative diagnostic criteria. Instead, these disorders are typically based on the absence of disconfirming evidence.

Differential Diagnosis

DSM-IV-TR recognizes six different diagnoses that might apply in cases of UMCs. These include FD, four of the five somatoform disorders (somatization disorder, conversion disorder, pain disorder, and hypochondriasis), and malingering.

According to DSM-IV-TR, the intentional and conscious production of symptoms must be established to diagnose FD and must be ruled out to diagnose a somatoform disorder. The nature of these determinations makes it relatively easy to diagnose the most severe cases of FD, but much more difficult to diagnose the least severe cases. For severe cases of FD in which there is clear evidence of organic pathology (e.g., festering wounds) requiring long hospital stays, affirmative evidence might be available from laboratory tests, room searches, or fortuitous direct observation. These may show that the patient has played an active role in producing his or her signs and symptoms. However, even in these cases, intentionality is more likely to be inferred through a painstaking process of diagnostic and treatment procedures that confirm the absence of any naturally occurring disease process that can account for the observed physical problem.

In cases characterized by UMCs for which there are no physical indicators (e.g., chronic pain or weakness), it is nearly impossible to confidently diagnose FD. To do so requires that the physician first confirm the absence of any medical problems that could adequately account for the patient's complaints. After all conceivable medical explanations are ruled out, the physician must determine whether the patient intentionally lied or misled medical staff. Because of the subjective nature of the patient's complaints, there is no way to "catch" him or her in a deception, as might be possible with a patient who is intentionally aggravating a wound.

This analysis raises an interesting predicament for the diagnosis of somatoform disorders. A correct diagnosis of a somatoform disorder requires the clinician to rule out FD. However, we can find no scientific evidence to support the ability of clinicians to affirmatively determine that a UMC is unconsciously produced. In reality, the decision that a UMC is unconsciously produced is based solely on the absence of proof that it is intentionally created or enacted.

Once it has been determined that the signs and symptoms have been produced intentionally, the diagnosis of FD requires that the clinician rule out malingering. To do so, the clinician must confirm the absence of financial, social, or legal motives that could account for the patient's sick role behavior. Persons who are sick routinely receive various rewards (e.g., gifts, liability settlements) and dispensations (e.g., excused absences from school or work); therefore, the clinician must determine whether the available incentives are sufficient to explain the patient's sick role behavior. Adding to the challenge, a patient's misrepresentations can stem from multiple incentives, both internal and external, that vary over time and even coexist. For instance, a patient may feign severe pain both to acquire opioids and to obtain nurturance from a solicitous nursing staff (Feldman and Ford 1999).

The nosological problems described previously are reflected in research on the reliability and usefulness of FD and related diagnoses (Freyberger and Schneider 1994). Inter-rater reliability for the general category of ICD-10 psychosomatic disorders is lower than the average inter-rater reliability estimate for all mental disorders. Among the psychosomatic disorders, FD has the lowest inter-rater agreement (Jantschek et al. 1995). In a German-speaking sample, the inter-rater agreement for FD was 0.33, compared with an overall agreement of 0.79 for all adult psychological disorders (Dittmann et al. 1996; Muhs and Ori 1995). In a study of the stability of various diagnoses within a 2-year period, Daradkeh et al. (1997) reported that FD had the lowest index of stability of all disorders studied. Analysis of the somatoform disorders has also produced disconcerting results (Skre et al. 1991).

Comorbidity

Further evidence of the overlap among FD and related disorders is their high comorbidity (Ford 1995). For example, Fink (1992a) reported that 20% of patients who fit the diagnosis of somatization disorder had previously been admitted for a problem determined to be factitious. Hypochondriasis is also found frequently to coexist with somatization disorder (Barsky et al. 1992). Several studies suggest that these disorders, particularly conversion disorder, somatization disorder, and factitious disorder, are more alike than different (Ford 1995; Jonas and Pope 1985). Each has a high comorbidity with anxiety, depression, and substance abuse; all occur more in women than in men; all begin in adolescence or early adulthood; and all tend toward a chronic course, though there may be periods of remission. Also, comorbidity with personality disorders is almost invariable in factitious disorder. Borderline personality disorder has been most consistently reported in Munchausen syndrome and factitious disorder as a whole (Kapfhammer et al. 1998a). According to DSM-IV-TR, if the patient's symptoms meet criteria for both personality disorder and factitious disorder, Axis I and Axis II diagnoses may be made concurrently.

Several commentaries have called for changes in the way FD and related disorders are approached, both from a clinical and a research standpoint (Kirkmayer and Robbins 1991; Mayou et al. 1995). Nadelson (1979, 1985, 1996) suggested that these disorders represented points on a continuum of chronicity, severity, and consciousness. Jonas and Pope (1985) also advocated a view of these disorders as a single entity, but specifically warned against relying on clinical evaluations of awareness and consciousness to make clinical judgments about the presence or absence of a specific somatoform disorder. Eisendrath (1996a) argued specifically for a continuum of factitious illness behavior. In our view, there may be much to be gained by abandoning the categorical approach to FD and related disorders in favor of a continuum approach. This way of thinking about UMCs may shift the attention of clinicians and researchers to the various underlying psychological processes that are responsible for the diverse array of UMCs.

Etiology

We have already discussed the limitations in the empirical evidence related to etiology. However, adventuresome clinicians have offered their own etiologic proposals, and these may have great utility in some cases.

The behavioral literature suggests that FD is the result of past social learning and current positive and negative reinforcement (Barsky et al. 1992; Schwartz et al. 1994). Patients with FD may have experienced a critical illness as a child or had a relative who was seriously ill. This experience of assuming the sick role, or of having a model who assumed the sick role, may be positively reinforced when the child experiences or witnesses the sympathy, attention, encouragement, and affection that is accorded occupants of the sick role. In addition, the sick role behavior may be negatively reinforced by an avoidance of responsibilities and duties.

Factitious illness behavior has also been viewed as the result of faulty cognitive processing (Croyle and Skelton 1991; Mechanic and Angel 1987). In this view, the actual illness behavior is seen as secondary to the patient's abnormal perceptions of bodily sensations (Barsky et al. 1996). This cognitive model suggests that the patient's perceptual deficits cause him or her to experience normal bodily functions as noxious or unusually intense, or to misinterpret normal physiological functions as alarming or dangerous. In the cognitive processing model, it is assumed that FD is ultimately guided by the patient's need to be reassured about his or her health. By frequently visiting physicians and undergoing physical examinations and procedures, the patient is reassured, albeit temporarily, that no health problems exist.

Psychodynamic theories of FD have a long history. As early as 17 years before the term "Munchausen syndrome" was introduced (Asher 1951), Menninger (1934) advanced the notion of "polysurgical addiction." Menninger postulated psychodynamic underpinnings to this variant of factitious behavior that were characterized by intense aggression toward oneself and the physician, the latter representing the "perceived sadistic parent." Incorporated into this formulation is the concept of a "compromise formation," in which a part of the body may need to be sacrificed to save the whole (i.e., the sense of self) and to avert suicide. Spiro (1968) suggested that early deprivation and trauma, weak self-identity, and superego deficits were etiologic. Other etiologic hypotheses have involved gratification of dependency needs; establishment of a well-defined role (i.e., the role of patient) to be played to forestall a decline in reality testing; achievement of a sense of mastery for patients who feel weak and vulnerable; and masochism, because such patients seek out situations that mix caring with pain (Ford 1996; Spivak et al. 1994). In general, therefore, current psychodynamic conceptualizations treat FD as an intrapsychic defense. This defense is mobilized in one of two ways: 1) as an outlet for sexual, aggressive, or oral drives or 2) as a means of protecting the ego from guilt or low self-esteem. In the first way, when experiences cause anger and hostility toward others, somatic complaints are used to elicit help and attention from others. The person then has the opportunity to reject the help as insufficient, thereby discharging the anger and reducing intrapsychic conflict (Barsky and Klerman 1983). In the second way, when a person is believed to be sick, he or she is excused from responsibilities and awarded sympathy, attention, and support. The illness becomes an excuse for failure and protects the ego from guilt and low self-esteem.

Although the behavioral, cognitive, and psychodynamic perspectives contribute to our understanding of factitious illness behavior, they cannot fully explain why people feign illness. The behavioral approach states that the sick role is desirable because it is positively or negatively reinforced through social learning. However, Schwartz, et al. (1994) found that social learning did not predict high health care utilization, a prominent behavior in most patients with FD. The cognitive theories are well tested and may be particularly useful in explaining hypochondriacal problems as a misinterpretation of bodily cues. However, in FD, physiological symptoms are not being misperceived or misinterpreted, they are being consciously produced. The implicit motivational assumption in the cognitive model is that people engage in illness behavior to ensure good health, but patients with severe FD are actually harming themselves and putting their health at risk. The psychodynamic explanations sometimes are compelling in the more severe cases of FD, but they remain largely untested.

A more recent proposal—one also requiring additional testing—was put forth by Hamilton and Janata (1997). They proposed a self-enhancement model of FD, suggesting that FD is often a means of increasing or protecting self-esteem in an attempt to compensate for unsatisfactory self-definitions. The authors stated that FD enhances or protects self-esteem through four possible pathways:

1. FD protects self-esteem by allowing patients to blame potential failure on their illness.
2. FD patients may receive a boost to their self-esteem through their associations with prestigious physicians and medical facilities.
3. FD gives patients a way to present themselves as heroic and brave or as medically knowledgeable and sophisticated. This proposed pathway is supported by the fact that as society begins to view patients with a particular disease more sympa-

thetically, the disease becomes more frequently seen in FD cases, a trend seen recently with cancer and AIDS (Baile et al. 1992; Zuger and O'Dowd 1992).

4. Receiving a diagnosis of a rare medical condition may allow FD patients to feel unique. This hypothesis is consistent with the fact that the disorders feigned by FD patients are often unusual or presented in a dramatic manner.

Biologically, there have been no genetic studies, though factitious disorders can be multigenerational within families (Goodwin 1988; Libow 2000). Brain imaging, neuropsychological testing, and electroencephalographic studies of these patients have been small in scale, and abnormalities observed in a minority of the patients are nonspecific (Feldman and Ford 1999).

Management

Before suggestions for managing FD are offered, it must be understood that the most important issue in the diagnosis and treatment of FD is early detection to prevent the increased suffering and risk associated with self-harm and unnecessary tests and procedures. It is also likely that patients in the early stages of FD are more amenable to psychiatric intervention.

Confrontation Versus Nonconfrontation

In the past, cases of FD were managed with strong confrontation. The physician discovering the fraud would directly address the patient, sometimes harshly, pointing out evidence of the deceptions and misappropriation of time, attention, and other resources. This approach rarely worked to change the patient's behavior. In fact, because the approach threatened the person's identity as a patient, it is likely that the person increased the severity of his or her illness and presented to another physician in an attempt to hold on to the purloined sick role (Lipsitt 1996; van der Feltz-Cornelis 2000).

The clinical approach then evolved into an approach in which the patient is confronted in a nonaggressive, nonpunitive way (Kellner and Eth 1982; Marriage et al. 1988; van Moffaert 1991).

Even while unmasking the patient's factitious behavior, the attending physician—often with a psychiatrist—redefines the behavior as a cry for help. Interestingly, this stance allows the patient to maintain the status of patient, albeit a psychiatric one, which is a role less valued by these patients and society as a whole. Paradoxically, in being shown not to have a medical illness, the patient is proved to have a psychiatric illness. Though this "softer" approach seems to be more successful than heavy-handed confrontation in case reports (e.g., Feldman and Duval 1997), the approach has mostly been unsuccessful as well (e.g., Stone 1977). It is possible that persons with subclinical levels of FD may be less threatened by a nonpunitive confrontation, but there is no evidence that such attempts have been made or have been successful.

These disappointing outcomes have stimulated further thinking about nonconfrontational approaches (Eisendrath 1989; Louis et al. 1985). Silver (1996) outlined suggestions for the treatment of conversion disorder, which may be quite helpful in treating FD as well. Silver suggested avoiding direct confrontation with patients and avoiding implications that their problems are strictly psychological, an approach also advocated by Servan-Schreiber et al. (2000a, 2000b) for treatment of patients with somatization disorder. Silver also supported behavioral shaping techniques, many of which are advocated by Eisendrath and Feder (1996) for the management of FD.

For a nonconfrontational approach to be successful, it must offer patients a way out, a way to "recover" from their illness without admitting their role in its cause. This step is accomplished by offering a rationale for recovery. For example, Eisendrath (1989) suggested teaching the patient techniques such as self-hypnosis that will ostensibly increase blood flow to wounds that are slow to heal. Rather than being exploited for any intrinsic value, self-hypnosis is used as a maneuver that allows the patient to relinquish the factitious behavior while saving face. In a parallel way, biofeedback has been used to provide a face-saving explanation for improvement in patients with nonepileptic seizures (Klonoff et al. 1983). Eisendrath (1989) also advocated the double bind as a strategy for treatment of FD. In the double bind, physicians clearly explain their expectations for recovery and inform the patient that if his or her condition does not improve, they will be forced to conclude that the problem is likely to be factitious in origin.

While using face-saving strategies, it is important that the reinforcements surrounding the patient's illness behavior remain consistent with the goals of recovery. The ultimate goal of recovery should be broken down into small attainable goals, and every small success should be reinforced with praise and encouragement. In addition, demonstrations of continued disability must not be reinforced. Such advice may be assumed, but it is of utmost importance that all professionals working with the patient (e.g., physicians, nurses, physical therapists, home health workers) give the patient a consistent explanation for the illness, expectation for recovery, and reinforcement only for "well" behaviors. In addition, efforts should be made to encourage nonprofessional caregivers, family members, and friends to do the same.

In a clear example of a behavioral approach for treatment of FD, Solyom and Solyom (1990) employed an operant conditioning approach that went beyond praise and encouragement for two patients with factitious paraplegia. Once the symptoms were determined to be factitious, the patients were told that electrical "faradic massage" would be used to "increase circulation and stimulate nerve endings" in their legs. They were told that if they did not respond to the initial treatment, the painful treatment would have to be lengthened. Both patients responded within 2 days and were able to walk within a week. They were then followed by a single physician and were able to maintain recovery for several years.

Biopsychosocial Model and Education

As patients are given face-saving options for recovery and reinforcement for success, it is important to gradually educate them about the interaction of mental and physical health. They should be helped to understand that physical health influences, and is influenced by, our psychological well-being as well as our social and cultural circumstances. Comorbid ailments such as mood or anxiety disorders should be treated pharmacologically in most cases (Earle and Folks 1986; Feldman and Escalona 1991; Folks 1995). Silver et al. (1986) referred to the biopsychosocial model of health and advocated teaching patients to understand that there is a multilevel system of health, disease, and treatment. The researchers found that explaining the role of stress in disease is a good place to start because, though individuals perceive stress as psychological, it can be readily explained in physiological terms. In fact, the connection between the patient's emotions and physiology is the core of a somatization management program known as the Personal Health Improvement Program. Clinicians using this approach have found that the concept of the "mind-body connection" has become well accepted by the public (Locke 1997). As patients come to understand and accept the biopsychosocial model, discussing the influence of psychological difficulties on their physical health will be met with much less resistance and defensiveness.

Maintenance of Progress Through Psychotherapy

Clinical experience and case reports suggest that nonconfrontational and behavioral techniques are the most useful strategies for the management of FD. However, if FD is truly a means of enhancing self-esteem and providing an identity for persons with poor self-esteem or self-worth, gains are not likely to be maintained until these issues are addressed.

In their work with patients with somatization disorder, Servan-Schreiber et al. (2000a, 2000b) recognized the difficulty in motivating patients to accept mental health interventions. They suggested that referring to therapy as "stress management for patients with chronic illness" may help ease patients into the mental health system. Therapy would involve exploration of alternative hobbies, activities, and accomplishments for which the person would be consistently reinforced. Alternatively, interpersonal and dynamic approaches could achieve the same goal by exploring the issues that seem to precipitate factitious illness behavior in particular patients (e.g., behavior associated with interpersonal conflict) and by helping the patient develop a more healthy sense of self. In addition, every individual has a "story," a way of defining himself or herself that is acceptable and appealing to others (White and Epston 1990). For the patient with FD, dramatic, intractable illnesses have become the story, with the individual playing the role of the brave, strong patient. Psychotherapy can help the patient rewrite the story in an adaptive way. Regardless of the therapeutic approach taken, the goal is the same: to offer alternative means of gaining the gratification that the sick role provided. This goal can also be met fortuitously. For instance, one woman with Munchausen syndrome, who was admitted approximately 800 times to hundreds of different hospitals throughout Europe, stopped the behavior only when she became responsible for the care of a pet cat in a hostel for the homeless. She knew that her readmission would lead to neglect of the animal by the other residents. Now viewing herself as a giver, not a recipient, of care, she ended the deceptions.

When FD is confirmed, clinicians should be aware of their own countertransference. As noted by Feldman and Feldman (1995, p. 379), "Both the patient's overt behaviors, such as actual bodily damage, and his or her underlying emotional issues can mobilize particularly intense reactions" in health professionals. Among these reactions are therapeutic nihilism, anger and aversion, nonemergent breaches of confidentiality, overidentification, and feelings of personal responsibility for the patient's ongoing behavior. The clinician will benefit from awareness of these feelings, and such insight will enhance the approach to the patient.

Once patients have decreased their inappropriate illness behaviors, it is important that their future medical care promotes appropriate patient behavior. It is often suggested that one physician coordinate all of the patient's medical services and that all physicians involved in the patient's care communicate clearly with one another. Physicians should realize that patients are likely to relapse in times of stress. If a safe, nonconfrontational relationship is established and the patient is educated according to the biopsychosocial model, there is a better chance that the patient will understand that the symptoms are a result of stress and will be open to psychological intervention.

Another avenue for prevention of future factitious symptoms is known as noncontingent medical care. In this approach, patients see their physicians regularly and therefore are not forced to fabricate symptoms to receive medical attention (Smith et al. 1986). The goal is to alter the contingencies of illness behavior through regularly scheduled appointments so that there is less advantage in feigning an illness. Schwarz et al. (1993) used a similar approach on an inpatient basis for one patient. The patient was allowed to admit and discharge herself from the hospital as she deemed necessary. This option allowed her to fulfill her needs for support without inducing illness in herself. After 1 year, her use of medical care decreased dramatically, until she eventually remained out of the hospital for at least 16 months.

It is unlikely that patients with FD will go through life without ever experiencing true health problems, making the management of FD all the more difficult. However, it is important that each of the patient's complaints is addressed at least briefly so that the patient is not required to exaggerate symptoms in order to receive medical care.

Conclusion

The existence of clear-cut cases of FD constitutes proof that there are persons who desperately want to garner the intangible, internal benefits of the sick role. Clinicians who attempt to assist patients with FD may find themselves frustrated by individuals who ostensibly present for definitive medical care but concurrently conceal the cause of the ailment, thus making definitive care impossible. Without an empirically validated set of affirmative criteria for determining the presence of FD or related disorders, physicians are left with no widely accepted standard of care for discontinuing the medical evaluation or treatment of these patients. The lack of affirmative diagnostic criteria means that these diagnoses can be made only after the medical staff has performed an exhaustive series of medical and surgical tests and treatments aimed at ruling out every conceivable pathology that might explain the patient's illness. Consequently, it may take many months, or even years, of negative medical findings before medical staff decide that the patient has been simulating or creating illness (Reich and Gottfried 1983). This understandably conservative approach to these patients is responsible for most of the costs outlined previously.

Notwithstanding the difficulties inherent in diagnosing FD under current nosological systems, it is almost certain that the underlying psychological processes that operate in the most blatant cases of FD are also at work in many more cases that are assigned a somatoform disorder diagnosis. This is also likely to be true in cases of UMCs that are never officially diagnosed. Effective early intervention in these cases will depend on the ability of clinical researchers to delineate these psychological processes and to develop assessment procedures to allow for the early diagnosis of FD. However, because there is virtually no empirical research on FD, there is no reliable source of information from which to develop a set of affirmative diagnostic criteria that would enable reliable early identification of these cases.

Little can be done about the reluctance of patients with FD to participate in research studies. As a result, the only way to collect information about FD and to explore issues such as etiology is through the reports of the physicians who encounter them. However, a method must be found to facilitate the reporting of more, and more representative, FD cases and to standardize the way these cases are presented. We believe that this can be done by creating a way for physicians to electronically register, via the Internet, cases of patients who they believe have exaggerated, feigned, or induced their own illness or injury. Using this strategy, any physician with Internet access, anywhere in the world, can register a case. For each case, the physician can supply information using a standardized reporting protocol, one that would include carefully selected psychosocial variables as well as demographic and medical history variables. One can only imagine how much more we would have been able to learn about FD if all of the published case reports of FD had been entered into a single database using a standardized reporting protocol.

Although reports of success in intervention in FD cases have been limited, a few overall management recommendations have surfaced. The approach should probably be nonconfrontational, offering the individual a face-saving means of recovery. In addition, a variety of behavioral techniques can be used to handle factitious symptoms and reinforce appropriate illness behavior. Education regarding the connection between mental and physical well-being has proven beneficial, and psychotherapy to help individuals attain identity and self-esteem more appropriately will probably be an important component of treatment for patients who will accept it. Maintaining healthy behaviors can be facilitated through brief but regularly scheduled medical office visits and recognition that patients may relapse in times of stress. Understanding that FD often serves the important function of providing self-esteem for individuals who otherwise have negative views of themselves may help clinicians intervene with these challenging, often disquieting, patients. As the self-enhancement model implies, these patients may abandon the sick role only when they have constructed alternative, healthier self-definitions.

References

Aduan RP, Fauci AS, Dale DD: Factitious fever and self-induced infection: a report of 32 cases and review of the literature. Ann Intern Med 90:230–242, 1979

American Psychiatric Association: Diagnostic and Statistical Manual of Mental Disorders, 4th Edition, Text Revision. Washington, DC, American Psychiatric Association, 2000

Asher R: Munchausen's syndrome. Lancet 1:339–341, 1951

Baile WF Jr, Kuehn CV, Straker D: Factitious cancer. Psychosomatics 33:100–105, 1992

Ballas SK: Factitious sickle cell acute painful episodes: a secondary type of Munchausen syndrome. Am J Hematol 53:254–258, 1996

Barsky AJ, Klerman GL: Overview: hypochondriasis, bodily complaints, and somatic styles. Am J Psychiatry 140:273–283, 1983

Barsky AJ, Wyshak G, Klerman GL: Psychiatric comorbidity in DSM-III-R hypochondriasis. Arch Gen Psychiatry 49:101–108, 1992

Barsky AJ, Ahern DK, Bailey ED, et al: Predictors of persistent palpitations and continued medical utilization. J Fam Pract 42:465–472, 1996

Bauer M, Boegner F: Neurological syndromes in factitious disorder. J Nerv Ment Dis 184:281–288, 1996

Bhugra D: Psychiatric Munchausen's syndrome. Literature review with case reports. Acta Psychiatr Scand 77:497–503, 1988

Bock KD, Overkamp F: Factitious disease. Observations on 44 cases at a medical clinic and recommendation for a subclassification [in German]. Klin Wochenschr 64:149–164, 1986

Bogazzi F, Bartalena L, Scarcello G, et al: The age of patients with thyrotoxicosis factitia in Italy from 1973 to 1996. J Endocrinol Invest 22: 128–133, 1999

Bridges KW, Goldberg DP: Somatic presentations of DSM-III psychiatric disorders in primary care. J Psychiatr Res 9:583–586, 1985

Bunim JJ, Federman DD, Black RL, et al: Factitious diseases: clinical staff conference at the National Institutes of Health. Ann Intern Med 48:1328–1341, 1958

Chua JD, Friedenberg WR: Superwarfarin poisoning. Arch Intern Med 158:1929–1932, 1998

Churchill DR, De Cock KM, Miller RF: Feigned HIV infection/AIDS: malingering and Munchausen's syndrome. Genitourinary Medicine 70:314–316, 1994

Craven DE, Steger KA, La Chapelle R, et al: Factitious HIV infection: the importance of documenting infection. Ann Intern Med 121:763–766, 1994

Croyle RT, Skelton JA: Mental Representation in Illness and Health. New York, Springer-Verlag, 1991

Cunnien AJ: Psychiatric and medical syndromes associated with deception, in Clinical Assessment of Malingering and Deception. Edited by Rogers R. New York, Guilford Press, 1988, pp 13–33

Daradkeh TK, El Rufaie OEF, Younis YO, et al: The diagnostic stability of ICD-10 psychiatric diagnoses in clinical practice. European Psychiatry 12:136–139, 1997

Dickinson EJ, Evans TR: Cardiac Munchausen's syndrome. J R Soc Med 80:630–633, 1987

Dittmann V, Albus M, Grefe J: Disorders of adult personality and behaviour (F6). Results from the ICD-10 field trial of the Diagnostic Criteria for Research in German-speaking countries. Psychopathology 29:301–305, 1996

Donovan DM: Costs of factitious illness. Hospital and Community Psychiatry 38:571–572, 1987

Earle JR Jr, Folks DG: Factitious disorder and coexisting depression: a report of successful psychiatric consultation and case management. Gen Hosp Psychiatry 8:448–450, 1986

Eckhardt-Henn A: Factitious disorders and Munchausen's syndrome. The state of research [in German]. Psychother Psychosom Med Psychol 49:75–89, 1999

Eisendrath SJ: Factitious physical disorders: treatment without confrontation. Psychosomatics 30:383–387, 1989

Eisendrath SJ: Current overview of factitious physical disorders, in The Spectrum of Factitious Disorders. Edited by Feldman MD, Eisendrath SJ. Washington, DC, American Psychiatric Press, 1996a, pp 21–36

Eisendrath SJ: When Munchausen becomes malingering: factitious disorders that penetrate the legal system. Bulletin of the American Academy of Psychiatry and the Law 24:471–481, 1996b

Eisendrath SJ, Feder A: Management of factitious disorders, in The Spectrum of Factitious Disorders. Edited by Feldman MD, Eisendrath SJ. Washington, DC, American Psychiatric Press, 1996, pp 195–213

Eisendrath SJ, Rand DC, Feldman MD: Factitious disorders and litigation, in The Spectrum of Factitious Disorders. Edited by Feldman MD, Eisendrath SJ. Washington, DC, American Psychiatric Press, 1996, pp 65–81

Faguet RA: Munchausen syndrome and necrophilia. Suicide Life Threat Behav 10:214–218, 1980

Feldman MD: The costs of factitious disorders. Psychosomatics 35:506–507, 1994

Feldman MD: Factitious disorders and fraud. Psychosomatics 36:509–510, 1995

Feldman MD, Duval NJ: Factitious quadriplegia. A rare new case and literature review. Psychosomatics 38:76–80, 1997

Feldman MD, Eisendrath SJ (eds): The Spectrum of Factitious Disorders. Washington, DC, American Psychiatric Press, 1996

Feldman MD, Escalona R: The longing for nurturance. A case of factitious cancer. Psychosomatics 32:226–228, 1991

Feldman MD, Feldman JM: Tangled in the web: countertransference in the therapy of factitious disorders. Int J Psychiatry Med 25:389–399, 1995

Feldman MD, Ford CV: Patient or Pretender: Inside the Strange World of Factitious Disorders. New York, Wiley, 1994

Feldman MD, Ford CV: Factitious disorders, in Kaplan and Sadock's Comprehensive Textbook of Psychiatry, 7th Edition. Edited by Sadock BJ, Sadock VA. Baltimore, JB Lippincott Williams & Wilkins, 1999, pp 1533–1543

Feldman MD, Smith R: Personal and interpersonal toll of factitious disorders, in The Spectrum of Factitious Disorders. Edited by Feldman MD, Eisendrath SJ. Washington, DC, American Psychiatric Press, 1996, pp 175–194

Fink P: Physical complaints and symptoms of somatizing patients. J Psychosom Res 36:125–136, 1992a

Fink P: The use of hospitalizations by persistent somatizing patients. Psychol Med 22:173–180, 1992b

Fink P, Jensen J: Clinical characteristics of the Munchausen syndrome. A review and 3 new case histories. Psychother Psychosom 52:164–171, 1989

Fishbain DA, Goldberg M, Rosomoff RS, et al: More Munchausen with chronic pain. Clin J Pain 7:237–244, 1991

Folks DG: Munchausen's syndrome and other factitious disorders. Neurol Clin 13:267–281, 1995

Folks DG, Feldman MD, Ford CV: Somatoform disorders, factitious disorders, and malingering, in Psychiatric Care of the Medical Patient, 2nd Edition. Edited by Stoudemire A, Fogel BS, Greenberg DB. New York, Oxford University Press, 2000, pp 458–475

Ford CV: The Somatizing Disorders: Illness as a Way of Life. New York, Elsevier, 1983

Ford CV: Illness as a lifestyle. The role of somatization in medical practice. Spine 17(10 suppl):S338–S343, 1992

Ford CV: Dimensions of somatization and hypochondriasis. Neurol Clin 13:241–253, 1995

Ford CV: Lies! Lies!! Lies!!! The Psychology of Deceit. Washington, DC, American Psychiatric Press, 1996

Freyberger HJ, Schneider W: Diagnosis and classification of factitious disorder with operational diagnostic systems. Psychother Psychosom 62:27–29, 1994

Freyberger H, Nordmeyer JP, Freyberger HJ, et al: Patients suffering from factitious disorders in the clinico-psychosomatic consultation liaison service: psychodynamic processes, psychotherapeutic initial care and clinicointerdisciplinary cooperation. Psychother Psychosom 62:108–122, 1994

Friedl MC, Draijer N: Dissociative disorders in Dutch psychiatric inpatients. Am J Psychiatry 157:1012–1013, 2000

Gault MH, Campbell NR, Aksu AE: Spurious stones. Nephron 48:274–279, 1988

Gavin H: On Feigned and Factitious Diseases, Chiefly of Soldiers and Seamen, On the Means Used to Simulate or Produce Them, and On the Best Mode of Discovering Imposters. London, John Churchill, 1843

Gill GV: The spectrum of brittle diabetes. J R Soc Med 85:259–261, 1992

Goodwin J: Munchausen's syndrome as a dissociative disorder. Dissociation 1:54–60, 1988

Hamilton JC, Janata JW: Dying to be ill: the role of self-enhancement motives in the spectrum of factitious disorders. Journal of Social and Clinical Psychology 16:178–199, 1997

Hardie TJ, Reed A: Pseudologia fantastica, factitious disorder and im-postership: a deception syndrome. Med Sci Law 38:198–201, 1988

Jantschek G, Rodewig K, von Wietersheim J, et al: Concepts of psycho-somatic disorders in ICD-10: results of the Research Criteria Study. Psychother Psychosom 63:112–123, 1995

Jonas JM, Pope HG Jr: The dissimulating disorders: a single diagnostic entity? Compr Psychiatry 26:58–62, 1985

Joseph-Di Caprio J, Remafedi GJ: Adolescents with factitious HIV dis-ease. J Adolesc Health 21:102–106, 1997

Kapfhammer HP, Dobmeier P, Mayer C, et al: Conversion syndromes in neurology. A psychopathological and psychodynamic differentia-tion of conversion disorder, somatization disorder and factitious dis-order [in German]. Psychother Psychosom Med Psychol 48:463–474, 1998a

Kapfhammer HP, Rothenhausler HB, Dietrich E, et al: Artifactual disor-ders—between deception and self-mutilation. Experiences in consul-tation psychiatry at a university clinic [in German]. Nervenarzt 69: 401–409, 1998b

Kellner CH, Eth S: Code blue—factitious cyanosis. J Nerv Ment Dis 170:371–372, 1982

King BH, Ford CV: Pseudologia fantastica. Acta Psychiatr Scand 77:1–6, 1988

Kirkmayer LJ, Robbins JM (eds): Current Concepts of Somatization: Re-search and Clinical Perspectives. Washington, DC, American Psychi-atric Press, 1991

Klonoff EA, Youngner SJ, Moore DJ, et al: Chronic factitious illness: a behavioral approach. Int J Psychiatry Med 13:173–183, 1983

Knockaert DC, Vanneste LJ, Vanneste SB, et al: Fever of unknown origin in the 1980s. An update of the diagnostic spectrum. Arch Intern Med 152:51–55, 1992

Kroenke K, Mangelsdorff AD: Common symptoms in ambulatory care: incidence, evaluation, therapy, and outcome. Am J Med 86:262–266, 1989

Labott SM, Preisman RC, Popovich J, et al: Health care utilization of so-matizing patients in a pulmonary subspecialty clinic. Psychosomat-ics 36:122–128, 1995

Libow JA: Child and adolescent illness falsification. Pediatrics 105:336–342, 2000

Lipsitt DR: Introduction, in The Spectrum of Factitious Disorders. Edit-ed by Feldman MD, Eisendrath SJ. Washington, DC, American Psy-chiatric Press, 1996, pp xix–xxviii

Locke SE: Treating somatization: an update. Behavioral Health Management 17:22–24, 1997

Louis DS, Lamp MK, Greene TL: The upper extremity and psychiatric illness. J Hand Surg [Am] 10:687–693, 1985

Ludwigs U, Ruiz H, Isaksson H, et al: Factitious disorder presenting with acute cardiovascular symptoms. J Intern Med 236:685–690, 1994

Marriage K, Govorchin M, George P, et al: Use of an amytal interview in the management of factitious deaf mutism. Aust N Z J Psychiatry 22:454–456, 1988

Mayou R, Bass CM, Sharpe M: Treatment of Functional Somatic Symptoms. New York, Oxford University Press, 1995

McCahill ME: Somatoform and related disorders: delivery of diagnosis as first step. Am Fam Physician 52:193–204, 1995

Meagher DJ, Collins AG: The use of aliases by psychiatric patients. Psychopathology 30:324–327, 1997

Mechanic D, Angel RJ: Some factors associated with the report and evaluation of back pain. J Health Soc Behav 28:131–139, 1987

Menninger K: Polysurgery and polysurgical addiction. Psychoanal Q 4:173–199, 1934

Mohammed R, Goy JA, Walpole BG, et al: Munchausen's syndrome. A study of the casualty "Black books" of Melbourne. Med J Aust 143:561–563, 1985

Muhs A, Ori C: Concepts of neurotic and personality disorders in ICD-10: results of the Research Criteria Study. Psychother Psychosom 63:99–111, 1995

Nadelson T: The Munchausen spectrum: borderline character features. Gen Hosp Psychiatry 1:11–17, 1979

Nadelson T: False patients/real patients: a spectrum of disease presentation. Psychother Psychosom 44:175–184, 1985

Nadelson T: Historical perspectives on the spectrum of sickness: from "crock" to "crook," in The Spectrum of Factitious Disorders. Edited by Feldman MD, Eisendrath SJ. American Psychiatric Press, Washington, DC, 1996, pp 1–20

Newmark N, Adityanjee, Kay J: Pseudologia fantastica and factitious disorder: review of the literature and a case report. Compr Psychiatry 40:89–95, 1999

Pankratz L: Patients Who Deceive: Assessment and Management of Risk in Providing Health Care and Financial Benefits. Springfield, IL, Charles C Thomas, 1998

Papadopoulos MC, Bell BA: Factitious neurosurgical emergencies: report of five cases. Br J Neurosurg 13:591–593, 1999

Plewes JM, Fagan JG: Factitious disorders and malingering, in The American Psychiatric Press Textbook of Psychiatry, 2nd Edition. Edited by Hales RE, Talbott JA, Yudofsky SC. Washington, DC, American Psychiatric Press, 1994, pp 623–632

Pope HG Jr, Jonas JM, Jones B: Factitious psychosis: phenomenology, family history, and long-term outcome of nine patients. Am J Psychiatry 139:1480–1483, 1982

Powell R, Boast N: The million dollar man. Resource implications for chronic Munchausen's syndrome [see comments]. Br J Psychiatry 162:253–256, 1993

Rabins PV: Reversible dementia and the misdiagnosis of dementia: a review. Hospital and Community Psychiatry 34:830–835, 1983

Reich JD, Hanno PM: Factitious renal colic. Urology 50:858–862, 1997

Reich P, Gottfried LA: Factitious disorders in a teaching hospital. Ann Intern Med 99:240–247, 1983

Risse M, Weiler G, Jedamzik J: Case report of pathologic and criminal self injury [in German]. Arch Kriminol 189:77–82, 1992

Rumans LW, Vosti KL: Factitious and fraudulent fever. Am J Med 65: 745–755, 1978

Sabot JF, Bornet CE, Favre S, et al: The analysis of peculiar urinary (and other) calculi: an endless source of challenge. Clin Chim Acta 283: 151–158, 1999

Sansone RA, Weiderman MW, Sansone LA, et al: Sabotaging one's own medical care. Arch Fam Med 6:583–586, 1997

Sarwari AR, Mackowiak PA: Factitious fever: a modern update. Curr Clin Top Infect Dis 17:88–94, 1997

Schwartz SM, Gramling SE, Mancini T: The influence of life stress, personality, and learning history on illness behavior. J Behav Ther Exp Psychiatry 25:135–142, 1994

Schwarz K, Harding R, Harrington D, et al: Hospital management of a patient with intractable factitious disorder. Psychosomatics 34:265–267, 1993

Servan-Schreiber D, Kolb NR, Tabas G: Somatizing patients: part I. Practical diagnosis. Am Fam Physician 61:1073–1078, 2000a

Servan-Schreiber D, Tabas G, Kolb R: Somatizing patients: part II. Practical management. Am Fam Physician 61:1423–1428, 2000b

Silver F: Management of conversion disorder. Am J Phys Med Rehabil 75:134–140, 1996

Silver PS, Auerbach SM, Vishniavsky N, et al: Psychological factors in recurrent genital herpes infection: stress, coping style, social support, emotional dysfunction, and symptom recurrence. J Psychosom Res 30:163–171, 1986

Skre I, Onstad S, Torgersen S, et al: Higher interrater reliability for the Structured Clinical Interview for DSM-III-R Axis I (SCID-1). Acta Psychiatr Scand 84:167–173, 1991

Smith GR Jr, Monson RA, Ray DC: Psychiatric consultation in somatization disorder. A randomized controlled study. N Engl J Med 314: 1407–1413, 1986

Solyom C, Solyom L: A treatment program for functional paraplegia/ Munchausen syndrome. J Behav Ther Exp Psychiatry 21:225–230, 1990

Spiro HR: Chronic factitious illness. Munchausen's syndrome. Arch Gen Psychiatry 18:569–579, 1968

Spivak H, Rodin G, Sutherland A: The psychology of factitious disorders. A reconsideration. Psychosomatics 35:25–34, 1994

Stone MH: Factitious illness. Psychological findings and treatment recommendations. Bull Menninger Clin 41:239–254, 1977

Suresh TR, Srinivasan TN: Claimed simulation of insanity. A coping strategy in mania. Br J Psychiatry 157:603–605, 1990

Sutherland AJ, Rodin GM: Factitious disorders in a general hospital setting: clinical features and a review of the literature. Psychosomatics 31:392–399, 1990

van der Feltz-Cornelis CM: Confronting patients about a factitious disorder [in Dutch]. Ned Tijdschr Geneeskd 144:545–548, 2000

van Moffaert MM: Integration of medical and psychiatric management in self-mutilation. Gen Hosp Psychiatry 13:59–67, 1991

White M, Epston D: Narrative Means to Therapeutic Ends. New York, Norton, 1990

World Health Organization: International Statistical Classification of Diseases and Related Health Problems, 10th Revision. Geneva, World Health Organization, 1992

Zuger A, O'Dowd MA: The baron has AIDS: a case of factitious human immunodeficiency virus infection and review. Clin Infect Dis 14:211–216, 1992

Afterword

Katharine A. Phillips, M.D.

Although knowledge of the somatoform and factitious disorders is steadily increasing—and knowledge of some of them is advancing at a rapid pace—they clearly require further investigation. Currently, for example, there is little research that sheds light on the classification questions raised in several chapters. For example, should the somatoform disorders section of DSM-IV-TR be disbanded? If so, where do these disorders belong? Data on their etiology and pathogenesis are needed in order for their classification to more accurately reflect their relationship to one another and to other disorders.

Even more important, research on the somatoform and factitious disorders is needed to improve patient care. As the preceding chapters attest, these disorders can be unusually distressing, impairing, and difficult to treat. Further research is essential to elucidate effective pharmacologic and psychosocial treatments. In addition, some of the exciting developments in our field, such as advances in genetics and neuroimaging, need to be applied to these disorders. Such approaches may ultimately elucidate their etiology and pathophysiology, which in turn may lead to more effective treatments. Our understanding of these disorders has advanced considerably since the time of Hippocrates; however, much remains to be learned.

Index

*Page numbers printed in **boldface** type refer to tables.*

Clomipramine
    body dysmorphic disorder
        and, 82, 83, 86
    hypochondriasis and, 47, 56
Clonazepam, 55
Cognitive-behavioral therapy.
    See also Behavioral therapy;
    Cognitive therapy;
    Psychotherapy
    body dysmorphic disorder
        and, 84–85, 87
    hypochondriasis and, 33–35,
        39–41, **37, 38,** 45–49, 59
    somatization disorder and,
        18
Cognitive processing, and
    factitious disorder, 149–150
Cognitive restructuring, and
    body dysmorphic disorder,
    85
Cognitive theory, of factitious
    disorder, 151
Cognitive therapy, and
    hypochondriasis, **38,** 39–41,
    45–47. *See also* Cognitive-
    behavioral therapy
Cohen, M. E., 4
Communication, and conversion
    disorder, 110
Comorbidity, of psychiatric
    disorders
    body dysmorphic disorder
        and, 68, 72, 78
    conversion disorder and,
        114–115
    factitious disorder and,
        148–149, 154–155
    somatization disorder and, 6,
        17, 19–20
Complications, of body
    dysmorphic disorder, 72–73

Composite International
    Diagnostic Interview, 6
Compulsive behaviors, and body
    dysmorphic disorder, 71–72
Conflict resolution, and
    somatization disorder, 9
Confrontation, and management
    of factitious disorder,
    152–153
Consultation
    factitious disorder and
        medicolegal, 140
    factitious disorder and
        psychiatric, 142
    somatization disorder and
        psychiatric, 17
Conversion. *See also* Conversion
    disorder
    in DSM-I and DSM-II, 95
    somatization disorder and, 2,
        4, 5
Conversion disorder. *See also*
    Conversion
    clinical features of, 110–111
    clinical subtypes of, 97–101
    comorbidity and, 114–115, 148
    diagnostic criteria for, 95, **96,
        97,** 101–102
    differential diagnosis of,
        115–117
    epidemiology of, 111–114
    factitious disorder and, 148
    functions served by symptoms
        of, 109–110
    history of concept of, 101–106
    models of symptom
        generation, 106–109
    somatic symptoms of, 12–13
    treatment of, 117–121
Coping skills. *See* Relaxation
    therapy

Cosmetic surgery, and body dysmorphic disorder, 68

Costs, of factitious disorder, 145–146, 158

Countertransference, and factitious disorder, 156

Course, of body dysmorphic disorder, 73–74

Culture
body dysmorphic disorder and, 75
somatization disorder and, 6

Cyberchondria, 29

Defense mechanisms
factitious disorder and, 150–151
hypochondriasis and, 31
somatization disorder and, 9

Delusional disorder, somatic subtype, 55

Delusions, and body dysmorphic disorder, 70, 79, 82, 87

Demographic characteristics, of patients with body dysmorphic disorder, 69

Dependent personality disorder, 114

Depression. *See also* Major depression
body dysmorphic disorder and, 78–79, 80
conversion disorder and, 114
hypochondriasis and, 31
somatic symptoms and, 12, 20

Dermatology, and body dysmorphic disorder, 68, 86, 88

Desipramine, 82

Developmental model, of somatic symptoms, 1

Diabetes, and factitious disorder, 142

Diagnosis. *See also* Differential diagnosis; Evaluation; Misdiagnosis
of body dysmorphic disorder, 80–81
of conversion disorder, 95, **96, 97**
of factitious disorder, 133–134, 140, 142, 147–148, 157–158

Differential diagnosis. *See also* Diagnosis
conversion disorder and, 115–117
factitious disorder and, 146–148
hypochondriasis and, 30
pseudoseizures and, 101
somatization disorder and, 12–13

Disability, and body dysmorphic disorder, 73

Disease phobia, and hypochondriasis, 28

Dissociative disorders, and conversion disorder, 114, 117

Dissociative identity disorder (DID), 101

Doctor-patient relationship, and hypochondriasis, 28–29

Dosage, of serotonin reuptake inhibitors for body dysmorphic disorder, 86

Double bind, and management of factitious disorder, 153–154

DSM-I, and conversion, 95

DSM-II, and conversion, 95, 102

DSM-III
body dysmorphic disorder and, 68
conversion disorder and, 95
somatization disorder and, 4

DSM-III-R
  body dysmorphic disorder
      and, 68
  factitious disorder and, 133,
      134, 146
  somatization disorder and, 5
DSM-IV
  body dysmorphic disorder
      and, 67, 80
  conversion disorder and, 95
  somatization disorder and, 2, 5
DSM-IV-TR
  conversion disorder and, **96,**
      97, 101–102, 106, 109
  factitious disorder and, 139,
      148
  somatization disorder and, **3**
Dysfunctional thoughts, and
    hypochondriasis, 34
Dysmorphophobia, 67

Eating disorders, and body
    dysmorphic disorder, 79
Education. *See also*
    Psychoeducation
  management of factitious
      disorder and, 154–155, 159
  treatment of hypochondriasis
      and, 45, 46, 51–52
Ego, and hypochondriasis, 31
Egypt, and ancient medical texts,
    102, **103**
Electroconvulsive therapy
  body dysmorphic disorder
      and, 83
  hypochondriasis and, 55
Electroencephalograms (EEGs),
    and conversion disorder, 99,
    115
Epidemiologic Catchment Area
    (ECA) study, 7–8

Epidemiology. *See also* Preva-
    lence
  of conversion disorder, 111–114
  of somatization disorder, 7–8
Ethnographic research, on
    somatization disorder, 6
Etiology
  of body dysmorphic disorder,
      76
  of factitious disorder, 149–152
  of somatization disorder, 9–11
Evaluation, of patients with
    somatization disorder, 13–16.
    See also Diagnosis
Explanatory therapy, and
    hypochondriasis, **38,** 51
Exposure therapy
  body dysmorphic disorder
      and, 84–85
  hypochondriasis and, 35, **36,**
      37, 39, 47–48, 49

Face-saving strategies, and
    management of factitious
    disorder, 153, 154
Factitious disorder (FD)
  associated features of, 139–140
  chart review and indicators of,
      141
  clinical description of, 134–139
  comorbidity and, 148–149
  conversion disorder and,
      109–110, 117
  costs of, 145–146, 158
  critique of literature on,
      130–132
  definition of, 129
  diagnosis of, 133–134, 142,
      147–148, 157–158
  differential diagnosis of,
      146–148

Factitious disorder (FD)
(*continued*)
etiology of, 149–152
management of, 152–157,
158–159
methods of simulating or
inducing medical
conditions, 136–139
prevalence of, 140, 142–145
Family. *See also* Family studies
and family history
body dysmorphic disorder
and, 88
somatization disorder and, 20
Family studies and family
history. *See also* Family;
Patient history
of body dysmorphic disorder,
76
of conversion disorder,
113
of factitious disorder, 152
of somatization disorder, 9
Finland, and somatization
disorder, 11
Flor-Henry, P., 108
Fluoxetine, and hypochondriasis,
53, 55, 56, 57–58
Fluvoxamine
body dysmorphic disorder
and, 82, 86
hypochondriasis and, **53**,
56–57
Folks, D. G., 107
Follow-up studies. *See also*
Outcome; Prognosis
conversion disorder and, 113
hypochondriasis and, 41
Ford, C. V., 107
Freud, Sigmund, 2, 4, 31, **103**,
104, 105–106, 107

Galen, 102, **103**
Gender. *See* Men; Women
Genetic studies, of somatization
disorder, 9. *See also* Family
studies and family history
Grief-induced hypochondria, 29
Group therapy. *See also*
Psychotherapy
hypochondriasis and, 35, **37**,
39
somatization disorder and, 18
Guilt, and hypochondriasis, 32
Guislain, J., 27
Guze, S. B., 5, 106

Hallucinations, and conversion
disorder, 98
Haloperidol, 55
Hamilton Anxiety Rating Scale,
40
Harvard Health Plan, 18
Head injury, and conversion
disorder, 115
Health Attitude Survey, **15**, 16
Health care services. *See also*
Medical conditions and
medical history
factitious disorder and, 145–146
somatization disorder and, 8,
14, 16–17
Heightened Illness Concern
Diary, 45, 56
Hemianesthesias, 99
Hippocrates, 102, **103**
Hispanic Americans, and
somatization disorder, 8
History, of psychiatric concepts
body dysmorphic disorder
and, 67–68
conversion disorder and,
101–106

hypochondriasis and, 27–28
somatization disorder and, 2–6
Histrionic personality disorder,
114
Homework assignments, and
hypochondriasis, 39
Human costs, of factitious
disorder, 145–146
Hurwitz, T. A., 107–108
Hypnosis, and conversion
disorder, 119–121
Hypochondriasis
clinical features of, 28–31
differential diagnosis of, 13,
30
factitious disorder and, 148
history of concept of, 27–28
theoretical models and
treatment of, 31–43
treatment considerations for,
43–59
Hysteria
conversion disorder and,
101–106, 111
somatization disorder and, 2, 4

ICD-10 (World Health
Organization)
dissociative disorders and
conversion, 96
factitious disorder and, 134,
135, 148
somatization disorder and, 7
Illness Attitude Scale, 39, 45, 51
Illness Behavior Questionnaire,
15–16, 55
Imipramine, and
hypochondriasis, **53,** 55–56
Insight
body dysmorphic disorder
and, 70, 78, 85

hypochondriasis and, 29–30,
33–34
Insight-oriented psychotherapy,
and body dysmorphic
disorder, 85, 87
Internet
factitious disorder and, 158
hypochondriasis and, 29, 31
Interpersonal relationships, and
factitious disorder, 136
In vivo exposure, and
hypochondriasis, 47
Israel, and somatization disorder, 8

Janet, P., 67–68, 98, **103,** 106

Kardiner, A., 107
Kidney stones, and factitious
disorder, 142
Koro, 75
Kraepelin, E., 67

Laboratory tests, and factitious
disorder, 138–139
Learning theory, and
somatization disorder, 9–10
Life experiences, and
somatization disorder, 10–11
Lithium, 83
Ludwig, A. M., 108

Major depression. *See also*
Depression
body dysmorphic disorder
and, 68, 72
conversion disorder and, 114
somatization disorder and, 12,
13
Management, of factitious
disorder, 152–157, 158–159.
See also Treatment

Maudsley, H., 29
Media, and factitious disorders, 129
Medical conditions and medical history. *See also* Health care services; Patient history; Unexplained medical complaints (UMCs)
   factitious disorder and, 136–139, **141,** 149
   hypochondriasis and, 30
   somatization disorder and, 8, 10
Medical Outcomes Study 36-Item Short-Form Health Survey (SF-36), 73
Medieval period, and concept of conversion, 102–103
MEDLINE search, 130–131
Melancholic hypochondria, 27–28
Men, and body dysmorphic disorder, 74
Meningitis, and factitious disorder, 139
Menninger, K., 150
Mesmer, F. A., **103,** 104
Mind-body connection, and factitious disorder, 155
Misdiagnosis. *See also* Diagnosis
   of body dysmorphic disorder, 80–81
   of conversion disorder, 116–117
Morita, S., 48
Morselli, E., 67, 70
Motor symptoms, and conversion disorder, 97–98
Multiple sclerosis, and conversion disorder, 115

Multisomatoform disorder, 6, 7
Munchausen syndrome, 135–136, 148, 156. *See also* Factitious disorder
Muscle dysmorphia, 74

Narcoanalysis, and conversion disorder, 118–119
Neuroleptic medications, and body dysmorphic disorder, 83
Neurological disorders, and conversion disorder, 112, 114–115
Neuropsychological studies, of body dysmorphic disorder, 76, 77
New York State Psychiatric Institute, 43
Nonconfrontational approaches, to management of factitious disorder, 153–154
Noncontingent medical care, and factitious disorder, 156–157
Nonverbal techniques, and somatization disorder, 19

Obsessional form, of hypochondriasis, 34
Obsessive-compulsive disorder (OCD)
   body dysmorphic disorder and, 68, 72, 77–78
   hypochondriasis and, 30–31, 34–35, 55
Operant conditioning, and factitious disorder, 154
Outcome, of hypochondriasis, 29. *See also* Follow-up studies; Prognosis

Pain and pain disorder
    conversion disorder and, 99,
        117
    somatization disorder and, **13,**
        20
Panic attacks, and conversion
        disorder, 114
Panic disorder
    body dysmorphic disorder
        and, 81
    differential diagnosis of
        somatization disorder
        and, **13**
    somatic symptoms of, 12
    treatment of hypochondriasis
        and, 55
Parental Bonding Instrument, 76
Parents, and responses to
        childhood illness, 10
Pathophysiology, of body
        dysmorphic disorder, 76
Patient history, and
        hypochondriasis, 44. *See also*
        Family studies and family
        history; Medical conditions
        and medical history
Perley, M. G., 5
Personal Health Improvement
        Program, 155
Personality, and somatization
        disorder, 11
Personality disorders
    body dysmorphic disorder
        and, 72
    conversion disorder and, 114
    factitious disorder and, 136,
        148
Phantom Illness (Cantor 1996), 45
Phobias. *See* AIDS; Social phobia
Physical abuse, and somatization
        disorder, 10–11

Physicians, and treatment of
        somatization disorder, 16–17
Physiologic model, of
        hypochondriasis, 41–43
Pilowsky, I., 28
Pimozide, and body dysmorphic
        disorder, 55, 83
Polysymptomatic somatoform
        disorder, 6
Possession, and concept of
        conversion, 102–103
Posttraumatic stress disorder,
        and conversion disorder, 114
Prevalence. *See also*
        Epidemiology
    of body dysmorphic disorder,
        68–69
    of conversion disorder,
        111–112
    of factitious disorder, 140,
        142–145
    of somatization disorder, 7–8
Prevention, of factitious disorder,
        156–157
Primary Care Evaluation of
        Mental Disorder (PRIME-
        MD), 14–15
Primary gain, and conversion
        symptoms, 111
Primary hypochondriasis, 55–58
Prognosis. *See also* Follow-up
        studies; Outcome
    of conversion disorder, 114
Pseudoseizures, and conversion
        disorder, 99–101, 112
Psychoanalytic psychotherapy,
        and hypochondriasis, **36**
Psychodynamic theory
    factitious disorder and, 150, 151
    hypochondriasis and, 31–33
    somatization disorder and, 9

Psychoeducation, and body
dysmorphic disorder, 88.
See also Education
Psychogenic seizures, 100–101,
112
Psychological approach, to
treatment of
hypochondriasis, 33–34
Psychological costs, of factitious
disorder, 146
Psychometry, and somatization
disorder, **15**. *See also*
Questionnaires; Rating
instruments; Self-report
instruments
Psychopharmacology. *See also*
Side effects; Treatment
body dysmorphic disorder
and, 81–84
hypochondriasis and, 52–60
somatization disorder and,
19–20
Psychophysiology, of
hypochondria, 42
Psychosomatic disorders, 148.
See also Factitious disorder
Psychotherapy. *See also*
Cognitive-behavioral
therapy; Group therapy;
Supportive psychotherapy;
Treatment
conversion disorder and, 118
factitious disorder and,
155–157, 159
hypochondriasis and, 32–33,
36–38
somatization disorder and,
17–19
Psychotic disorders
body dysmorphic disorder
and, 81

conversion disorder and, 101,
117
factitious disorder and,
140
somatization disorder and, 12,
13
Purtell, J. J., 4

Quality of life, and body
dysmorphic disorder, 73
Questionnaires. *See also*
Psychometry
assessment of
hypochondriasis and, 40,
45
evaluation of somatization
disorder and, 14–16

Rating instruments, and
hypochondriasis, 51. *See also*
Psychometry
Rating Scale of Somatic
Symptoms, 51
Raulin, J., 103
Reassurance
hypochondriasis and, 52
somatization disorder and,
18–19
Recommendations
on pharmacologic treatment of
hypochondriasis, 59
on treatment strategies for
body dysmorphic
disorder, 86–88
Referential thinking, and body
dysmorphic disorder, 70
Referrals, for psychiatric care in
cases of somatization
disorder, 17
Reinforcement, and factitious
disorder, 154